THE SPORTS SUPPLEMENT BIBLE

For Health and Fitness

BY
Will Brink

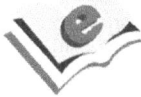

Internet-Publications.net

The Sports Supplement Bible: For Health and Fitness
Will Brink

Published By
Internet-Publications.net
P.O. Box 1892
Framingham, MA 01701
www.internet-publications.net

AUTHOR BIO

Will Brink is a columnist, contributing consultant, and writer for numerous health/fitness, medical, and bodybuilding publications. His articles on nutrition, supplements, weight loss, exercise and medicine can be found in magazines and journals such as "Muscle Insider", "Lets Live," "Muscle Media 2000," "MuscleMag International," "Life Extension," "Muscle & Fitness," "Inside Karate," "Exercise for Men Only," "Oxygen," "The Townsend Letter For Doctors," as well as many international magazines.

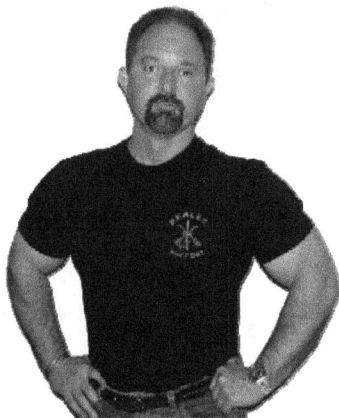

He is the author of the book "Priming The Anabolic Environment: A practical and Scientific Guide to the Art and Science of Building Muscle," as well as various chapters in sports nutrition related textbooks and is author of the e-books "Fat Loss Revealed" and "Brink's Bodybuilding Revealed."

Will graduated from Harvard University with a concentration in the natural sciences, and is a consultant to supplement companies. He has co-authored several studies relating to sports nutrition and health and published in peer reviewed academic journals.

He has served as an NPC judge and as a Ms. Fitness USA judge. A well-known trainer, Will has helped many top level bodybuilders through all facets of pre-contest and off-season training. He was an Adjunct Trainer at Smith & Wesson Training Academy and has written the book "Practical Applied Stress Training, for Tactical Law Enforcement", named after the class he taught. He has worked with athletes ranging from professional golfers, fitness contestants, and police and military personnel.

His articles and interviews can be found on many internet web sites such as: LEF.org, Testosterone.net, NavySeals.com, ThinkMuscle.com, MuscleMonthly.com, as well as many others, including his own site BrinkZone.com.

Will has lectured at trade associations and universities around the United States and has appeared on numerous radio and television programs to examine issues of health and fitness.

Warnings

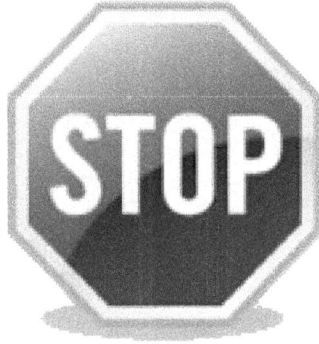

The instructions and advice presented should not be used as a substitute for medical or other personal professional counseling. This book is not intended to give medical advice or replace your doctor.

A basic metabolic test, thyroid, lipid, cardiovascular and testosterone panel is recommended prior to starting any program in order to detect anything that can prevent you from making the most out of your efforts. Consult your doctor regarding these tests.

You should speak with your doctor before taking any supplements as they can interfere with any medical therapies or cause problems if you have a medical condition.

CONTENTS AT A GLANCE

AUTHOR BIO 3

WARNINGS 5

HOW THIS BOOK WORKS 9

AMINO ACIDS 12

L–Arginine 14
Beta–Alanine 19
Branched Chain Amino Acids (BCAAs) 24
Citrulline 27
L–Glutamine 31
Ornithine Alpha–Ketoglutarate (OKG) 35
Taurine 40
L–Tyrosine 44

METABOLITES 47

Agmatine 49
Arachidonic Acid 54
Creatine Monohydrate 59
Carnitine 68
DHEA 72
7–Keto DHEA 76
GABA 80
HMB and KIC 85
Phosphatidylserine 90

RIBOSE 94

PROTEIN POWDERS 99

CASEIN 101
COLOSTRUM.. 108
EGG WHITE PROTEIN 112
SERUM PROTEIN ISOLATE... 115
VEGETARIAN PROTEINS: SOY, HEMP, RICE 120
WHEY PROTEIN 125

ESSENTIAL ELEMENTS 134

CALCIUM... 137
CHROMIUM PICOLINATE.. 140
ESSENTIAL FATTY ACIDS: INCLUDES FLAX, FISH AND OTHERS 143
FISH OIL 152
VANADYL SULPHATE 159
VITAMIN C 163
VITAMIN E 166
ZMA 170

ANTI-ESTROGENS 174

ATD... 176
CHRYSIN 181
I3C/DIM 184
6–OXO 188

HERBAL TESTOSTERONE BOOSTERS 192

AVENA SATIVA 194
FENUGREEK (TESTOFEN™).. 198
HORNY GOAT WEED 204
MACA... 209
RESVERATROL.. 212
TONGKAT ALI (LONG JACK)... 215
TRIBULUS TERRESTRIS 220
URTICA DIOICA 224

PHYTOCHEMICALS 227

BETA–SITOSTEROL.. 228
ECDYSTERONE 232
METHOXYISOFLAVONE 235

ADAPTOGENS 238

ASHWAGANDHA.. 239
BACOPA MONNIERI 243

CORDYCEPS 248
GINSENG 252
RHODIOLA ROSEA 256

MISCELLANEOUS COMPOUNDS 260

CAFFEINE 261
CISSUS QUADRANGULARIS 268
CHOCAMINE™ 272
CLA (CONJUGATED LINOLEIC ACID) 275
GH SUPPLEMENTS 280
GLYCEROL 286
MEDIUM CHAIN TRIGLYCERIDES (MCTs) 290
MYOSTATIN INHIBITORS 294
SAW PALMETTO 299

PROHORMONES & DESIGNER STEROIDS 307

MAKING SENSE OF SUPPLEMENTS 311

GAIN TWENTY POUNDS OF MUSCLE LOSE FIFTY POUNDS OF FAT! 311
THE SUPPLEMENT PYRAMID 313

THE SUPPLEMENT SCORECARD 320

FOUNDATIONAL SUPPLEMENTS 320
PERFORMANCE ENHANCEMENT SUPPLEMENTS 321
SUPPLEMENTS THAT ARE OPTIONAL, BUT CAN BE USEFUL FOR A MUSCLE
BUILDING PROGRAM 322
OTHER PROTEINS 323
SUPPLEMENTS TO EXPERIMENT WITH OR MIGHT BE WORTH A TRY 324
SUPPLEMENTS USEFUL FOR SPECIFIC APPLICATIONS 326
SUPPLEMENTS THAT ARE UNPROVEN OR INEFFECTIVE 327
USING THE SUPPLEMENT SCORECARD 329

FOR MORE INFORMATION 334

INFORMATION ON SUPPLEMENTS 334
STUDIES AND OTHER SCIENTIFIC DATA 334

INDEX 335

HOW THIS BOOK WORKS

There are literally thousands of supplements on the market from manufacturers and distributors around the world. When I first decided to write this book, I knew it would be impossible for me to review all of brand name supplements as any reviews I wrote would be rendered useless by changes in ingredients or recommended doses. And with new supplements constantly appearing on the market, this book would be obsolete within months.

This is why I focus on the ingredients in the supplements rather than the brand name supplements themselves. The vast majority of Over The Counter (or OTC) supplements are formulated from the same relatively short list of nutrients. By knowing the science behind the claims made for each compound, you can accurately predict whether a supplement containing those compounds is worth purchasing.

> An often used proverb goes *"Give a man a fish and you feed him for a day. Teach a man to fish and you feed him for a lifetime"*.

So with this type of approach, all of the bases are covered; reviews of specific brand name supplements AND nutrients/ingredients, using a format that can be constantly updated as new information comes in.

I put together this book in this manner to put the power of knowledge in your hands so that you can pick up any product and decide for yourself whether or not a particular brand name supplement is worth spending your hard earned money on.

While I'll not try to put you to sleep with overly technical jargon, I will cover the science – or lack there of – for those interested. Here's how I'll break up each review into easy to follow sections:

- ➢ **What is it?**
- ➢ **What is it supposed to do?**
- ➢ **What does the research have to say?**
- ➢ **What about real world athletic performance?**
- ➢ **Will Brink's Recommendation**

What is it? Gives a short overview of what the compound; what it is made of, where it comes from, and other information.

What is it supposed to do? Covers what a nutrient can or supposedly does and how it achieves the effect, assuming it has an effect.

What does the research have to say? Looks at actual published studies and give you an overview of the research on a particular nutrient or formula where applicable.

What about real world athletic performance? Tells you what people who have used the product have to say about their experiences. This section is a combination of the feedback I have received over the years from people I've worked with, as well as virtually thousands of emails and other 'net related discussions, and my own first hand experiences, which is over 30+ years worth now.

Will Brink's Recommendation Summarizes the potential pros and cons of all the sections and gives my no B.S. advice on whether a product is worth using.

Following the reviews, read the chapter **Making Sense of Supplements** which provides a framework for prioritizing and choosing supplements.

Also in this chapter, check out the supplement pyramid for an at-a-glance view of what is the most important part of your supplement arsenal.

The final chapter, **The Supplement Scorecard**, helps you to sum up all you've learned in this book, and helps you to pick out the most important ingredients in any supplement; allowing you to see if its actually worth taking.

To get more information along with the latest scientific data on supplements as they come out you can visit me at http://www.brinkzone.com.

For ongoing Q&A and discussion for this book in particular, go to http://sportssupplementbible.com

Chapter

1

AMINO ACIDS

A mino acids are the building blocks of protein. Our bodies break down the proteins we eat into individual amino acids and peptides, which are in turn are used to create the proteins we need to function. Proteins serve many different roles: structural, transport, catalysis, contraction, and protection against disease, to name only a few.

Amino acids are also involved in many non-protein reactions. Amino acids are used to

Amino Acids Covered

❖ **L–Arginine**

❖ **Beta–Alanine**

❖ **Branched Chain Amino Acids (BCAAs)**

❖ **Citrulline**

❖ **L–Glutamine**

❖ **Ornithine Alpha–Ketoglutarate (OKG)**

❖ **Taurine**

❖ **L–Tyrosine**

produce neurotransmitters, hormones, and other metabolites, such as creatine or citrulline. Amino acids may also be used as a source of energy.

- There are 20 amino acids that form most mammalian proteins. Each amino acid has a similar structure, but differ in the type of side chain attached to each α–carbon. The side chains confer different properties to each amino acid, and are responsible for the three-dimensional "native" structure of each protein. Amino acids are classified as essential, non-essential, or conditionally essential:

- Essential amino acids are those that our bodies cannot make, and must be supplied by the food we eat. There are 8 essential amino acids: methionine, leucine, valine, isoleucine, threonine, tryptophan, lysine, and phenylalanine. You may see the number listed as 9 or 10 in some places, as arginine and histidine are essential amino acids for infants and very young children.

- Non-essential amino acids can be produced by our bodies from other amino acids.

- Conditionally essential amino acids are non-essential amino acids that become essential under conditions of physical stress or trauma, when the body cannot produce a sufficient amount to meet demand. Some conditionally essential amino acids are: glutamine, arginine, cysteine and taurine. Not all amino acids are found in proteins. For example, both taurine and beta–alanine perform non-protein functions exclusively.

Note: I will not cover every amino acid in this section, only those that may have direct application to sports nutrition, performance, etc.

L–ARGININE

What is it?

Arginine is a conditionally essential amino acid. It's an essential amino acid in infancy/early childhood, and under stress conditions where the body cannot manufacture sufficient L–arginine to meet increased demand. Beyond its role in protein synthesis, arginine is a precursor for a number of important metabolites, including creatine and nitric oxide. It is an important intermediate in the urea cycle, and can stimulate the secretion of growth hormone.

What is it supposed to do?

The current interest in arginine and related compounds such as arginine–alpha–ketoglutarate (AAKG) lies in its role in the production of nitric oxide (NO). NO is the new superstar molecule with researchers as it appears to play a role directly or indirectly in almost every aspect of human physiology, such as the immune system, nervous system, circulatory system, and many others.

Arginine is a key component of the NO production pathway (arginine serves as the substrates for the nitric oxide synthase enzyme, which produces citrulline and NO from arginine) which is essential for a cascade of reactions involved in vasodilation and cardiovascular function.

Supplements containing arginine/AAKG are supposed to enhance the production of NO, and increase the "pump" you get during a hard workout in the gym.

What does the research say for athletic performance?

Recent data suggest arginine may have some legitimate uses regarding health and well-being. For example, the lining of artery walls called the endothelium needs to dilate and contract effectively.

NO is essential to this function and several studies have found arginine supplements at 8-20 grams per day restored endothelial vasodilation in the coronary arteries and may improves overall blood flow, which is important for people suffering from ischemic issues.

Another study suggested that arginine supplementation greatly improved penile function in men with penile dysfunction as NO is essential for blood flow involved in getting an erection.

Arginine has shown a very good safety profile to date and appears to have virtually no toxic effects. From an athletic/muscle building point of view, things become much less clear. Early studies suggested arginine could increase growth hormone levels, but in truth (a) these effects were found using very high doses and were intravenous and (b) short lived spikes in GH don't appear to have any positive effects on muscle mass or performance in healthy athletes anyway.

NO is a messenger molecule related to virtually every pathway in the human body, one way or another. Therefore, simply raising NO will have both positive and negative effects, most of which are not known at this time.

Having chronically elevated levels of NO above normal may not be a good idea. For example, though NO is associated with some potentially positive effects mentioned above, elevated NO levels are also associated with some negative effects. High levels of NO are associated with increased levels of an extremely powerful pro-oxidant called peroxynitrate, which immune cells use to kill pathogens. High levels of peroxynitrate may lead to greater oxidative stress, immune disorders, and increased inflammation. For example, high levels of NO and peroxynitrate are associated with fibromyalgia, chronic fatigue, and multiple chemical sensitivity. Therefore, it might not be a wise idea to have chronically elevated levels, especially if you have any of the aforementioned syndromes.

What about real world athletic performance?

A decade ago, arginine had a brief day in the limelight with athletes as a supplement that might stimulate growth hormone. However, its use as a GH releaser never materialized into new muscles for users, so it quickly fell out of favor.

Recently, however, there has been a resurgence of interest in arginine by athletes and supplement companies. This is due to recent findings showing a long list of possible uses with arginine, ranging from possible protection from heart disease, reducing cholesterol, to increasing blood flow.

This brings us to the new supplements known as "hemodilators" that claim to give you a "perpetual pump" and other marketing buzz words based on elevated NO. These new products are based on a form of arginine called Arginine Alpha–Ketoglutarate, which is simply arginine bound to alpha keto glutarate (AKG), a supplement that had a short life some years ago. Some of these new supplements claim some form of time delay or extended release to keep NO elevated.

There are many problems with the above, some of which I have mentioned already.

For one thing, there are no data to show such products keep NO elevated all day, there may be medical and physiological reasons to avoid constantly elevated levels of NO, and there are no studies at all showing such products increase LBM. In fact, there's even been one study that demonstrates that NO supplements are worthless for increasing LBM.

One study, sponsored by an NO supplement manufacturer, concluded:

" A AKG supplementation appeared to be safe and well tolerated, and positively influenced 1RM bench press and Wingate peak power performance. AAKG did not influence body composition or aerobic capacity."

To say that supplement manufacturers are overstating the muscle building effects of these new (and they are not really new, but are just being repackaged as new) products is being kind...

Interestingly, while some improvements in performance were seen in the prior study, these may well be due to the age of the subjects being tested in both studies: 30–50 year old men. Middle aged men are more likely to have some markers of cardiovascular disease, such as elevated homocysteine and asymmetrical dimethylarginine (ADMA) levels. ADMA is a competitive inhibitor of nitric oxide synthase (NOS), which is the enzyme responsible for NO production.

So positive performance results in this group may be due to a reduction in ADMA inhibition of NOS, rather than to the increased availability of arginine for NO production. Under normal conditions, arginine is not limiting for NO production, so increasing arginine should not result in increased NO production.

It's important to note, a variety of recent studies have found no increases in blood flow to muscles, nor increases in protein synthesis, or changes in other markers that would indicate benefit to athletes, with arginine.

Will Brink's Recommendation

From a health perspective, arginine and arginine alpha–ketoglutarate, may have some real uses for people with high cholesterol, coronary artery disease, ischemic (meaning a reduced blood flow and oxygen delivery to tissues) and even men with erectile dysfunction. As for athletes, the jury is still out for either arginine or arginine alpha–ketoglutarate.

Bottom line, I would not recommend them to athletes at this time for increasing either muscle mass or performance. For that use, they get a thumbs down.

References

Bloomer, R. Nitric Oxide Supplements for Sports Strength & Conditioning Journal: April 2010 - Volume 32 - Issue 2 - pp 14-20.

Tang JE, Lysecki PJ, Manolakos JJ, Macdonald MJ, Tarnopolsky MA, Phillips SM. Bolus Arginine Supplementation Affects neither Muscle Blood Flow nor Muscle Protein Synthesis in Young Men at Rest or After Resistance Exercise. J Nutr. 2010 Dec 29.

Campbell B, Roberts M, Kerksick C, et al. Pharmacokinetics, safety, and effects on exercise performance of L–arginine alpha–ketoglutarate in trained adult men. Nutrition. 2006 Sep;22(9):872–81.

Pall ML. Elevated, sustained peroxynitrite levels as the cause of chronic fatigue syndrome. Medical Hypotheses 2000;54:115–125.

Pall ML. Common etiology of posttraumatic stress disorder, fibromyalgia, chronic fatigue syndrome and multiple chemical sensitivity via elevated nitric oxide/peroxynitrate. Med Hypoth 2001;57:139–145.

Pall ML. Cobalamin used in chronic fatigue syndrome therapy is a nitric oxide scavenger. J Chronic Fatigue Syndr 2001:8(2);39–44.

ቀ

BETA–ALANINE

What is it?

Beta–alanine is the only naturally occurring beta amino acid. Beta amino acids have their primary amino groups attached to the beta, rather than the alpha carbon. Although beta–alanine is involved in the formation of other, larger molecules, it is not found in proteins.

What is it supposed to do?

Beta–alanine is being touted as "the new creatine" and the latest breakthrough supplement in the world of sports nutrition. It's used by the body to synthesize carnosine (L–beta–alanyl–L–histidine). Carnosine performs a variety of valuable roles, including: inhibiting the formation of advanced glycation end products (AGEs) which can damage tissues, chelating metal ions, and scavenging free radicals. Carnosine's importance to athletic performance, however, lies in its ability to buffer hydrogen ions produced in skeletal muscle during high intensity exercise.

So why not just use carnosine you ask? Though you will find more in depth information below, here's the reason in a nutshell: Studies show ingested carnosine is simply broken down into its constituent parts and reformed into carnosine. Studies generally find that ingesting beta–alanine is actually superior for increasing tissue carnosine levels then ingesting carnosine itself. More detail to follow…

What does the research say for athletic performance?

An increase in muscle carnosine appears to be an adaptation to resistance training. One recent study discovered that carnosine concentration in the skeletal muscle of competitive bodybuilders was twice that of controls. The researchers noted that the amount of carnosine measured represented 20% of the total buffering capacity of the muscle and stated:

" The increase in buffering capacity could influence the ability to carry out intense muscular activity."

So increasing carnosine in skeletal muscle has the potential to improve performance. In spite of this, it's unclear if direct supplementation with carnosine will have this effect. Studies are limited on the effects of carnosine supplementation on performance. From what little there is, there does not appear to be any benefit. This may be due to the fact that oral carnosine is broken down by intestinal and plasma carnosinases before significant amounts can be taken up into skeletal muscle.

Recent research indicates that supplying the carnosine precursor, beta–alanine, may be a far more effective means of increasing muscle carnosine stores. One recent study demonstrated that beta–alanine supplementation increased carnosine in the vastus lateralis by nearly 60% after 4 weeks, and 80% after 10 weeks. In addition, the researchers found that the total work done (TWD)—as measured by a cycling capacity test—improved with supplementation:

" ...4 wks beta–alanine supplementation resulted in a significant increase in TWD(+13.0%); with a further +3.2% increase at 10 wks. TWD was unchanged at 4 and 10 wks in the control subjects. The increase in TWD with supplementation followed the increase in muscle carnosine."

Does beta–alanine supplementation improve performance? Very recent research suggests that it might. One study on untrained men found that 28 days of beta–alanine supplementation delayed the onset of neuromuscular fatigue on a contiunous cycle ergometry test. A similar study in women confirmed increases of 13.9%, 12.6% and 2.5% for ventilatory threshold, physical working capacity at fatigue threshold, and time to exhaustion. A third study on 55 men suggested that a combination of beta–alanine and creatine monohydrate improved endurance performance.

Newer studies are suggestive of benefit, but how beneficial is still unclear. For example, one recent study gave trained collegiate wrestlers and football players 4g per day of beta-alanine using a double blind placebo testing protocol, and although there were improvements in strength and body mass in the group receiving the supplement, the authors found

"Although not statistically significan t(p > 0.05) subjects taking β–alanine achieved more desirable results on all tests compared to those on placebo."

What about real world athletic performance?

Beta–alanine is still a fairly new supplement and requires more extensive research, but "on paper" looks promising so far. Users feel that it helps with recovery and soreness, although the jury is still out whether it actually improves performance or—indirectly—LBM.

This supplement might be especially useful for vegetarians or people who eat limited amounts of meat, as meat is a primary source of dietary carnosine/beta–alanine.

Will Brink's Recommendations

With all that we know about the benefits of carnosine, I give this supplement two thumbs up for anyone interested in general health and well-being. More research needs to be done before it can be recommended as a performance enhancer, but is certainly worth a try, so I will give it a thumbs up as a supplement worth a shot and a supplement to keep an eye out for as additional studies come in.

Although studies are limited as to what the optimal dose is, 3-6 g/day appears to be an effective dose. So, If you see a few hundred milligrams in a product, it's probably worthless.

References

Kern BD, Robinson TL,. Effects of β–alanine supplementation on performance and body composition in collegiate wrestlers and football players. J Strength Cond Res. 2011Jul;25(7):1804-15.

Gardner ML, Illingworth KM, Kelleher J, Wood D. Intestinal absorption of the intact peptide carnosine in man, and comparison with intestinal permeability to lactulose. J Physiol. 1991 Aug;439:411-22.

Guiotto A, Calderan A, Ruzza P, Borin G. Carnosine and carnosine–related antioxidants: a review. Curr Med Chem. 2005;12(20):2293-315. Harris RC, Tallon MJ, Dunnett M, et al. The absorption of orally supplied beta–alanine and its effect on muscle carnosine synthesis in human vastus lateralis. Amino Acids. 2006 May;30(3):279-89.

Hill CA, Harris RC, Kim HJ, Harris BD, et al. Influence of beta–alanine supplementation on skeletal muscle carnosine concentrations and high intensity cycling capacity. Amino Acids. 2006 Jul 28.

Hipkiss AR. Glycation, ageing and carnosine: are carnivorous diets beneficial? Mech Ageing Dev. 2005 Oct;126(10):1034-9.

Park YJ, Volpe SL, Decker EA. Quantitation of carnosine in human plasma after dietary consumption of beef. J Agric Food Chem. 2005 Jun 15;53(12):4736-9.

Stout JR, Cramer JT, Mielke M, O'Kroy J, et al. Effects of twenty-eight days of beta–alanine and creatine monohydrate supplementation on the physical working capacity at neuromuscular fatigue threshold. J Strength Cond Res. 2006 Nov;20(4):928-31.

Stout JR, Cramer JT, Zoeller RF, Torok D, et al. Effects of beta–alanine supplementation on the onset of neuromuscular fatigue and ventilatory threshold in women. Amino Acids. 2007 Apr;32(3):381-6.

Tallon MJ, Harris RC, Boobis LH, et al. The carnosine content of vastus lateralis is elevated in resistance–trained bodybuilders. J Strength Cond Res. 2005 Nov;19(4):725-9.

Zoeller RF, Stout JR, O'kroy JA, Torok DJ, et al. Effects of 28 days of beta–alanine and creatine monohydrate supplementation on aerobic power, ventilatory and lactate thresholds, and time to exhaustion. Amino Acids. 2006 Sep 5.

φ

BRANCHED CHAIN AMINO ACIDS (BCAAS)

What are they?

The branch chain amino acids (so named because they branch off another chain of atoms rather than form a straight line as other amino acids do) are leucine, valine and isoleucine.

What are they supposed to do?

BCAAs are supposed to enhance lean mass gains by a) reducing muscle catabolism; and b) stimulating the synthesis of muscle protein.

What does the research say for athletic performance?

The BCAAs are the amino acids that are primarily used (oxidized) during exercise and make up to one third of the amino acids in muscle tissue. It has been known for a long time that BCAAs play a critical role in the turnover of lean body tissues (muscle) and is muscle sparing (i.e. anti-catabolic) in a variety of muscles wasting states. Of the three BCAAs, L–leucine appears to be the most important to preserve hard earned muscle mass; intense exercise and certain disease states have been shown to eat up a great deal of L–leucine.

So far so good! On the research front, some studies have found the consumption of BCAA before endurance exercise may decrease the rate of protein degradation and may have a sparing effect on muscle glycogen degradation, and depletion of muscle glycogen stores.

However, leucine supplementation at 200 mg per kg of body weight prior to anaerobic running exercise (sprinting) did not improve performance. Truth is, research to date with BCAAs and performance has been contradictory, at best. One of the major drawbacks of the BCAAs as a supplement is dosage.

It takes very high doses to see any ergogenic effect, assuming there are any ergogenic effects to be had, as studies are still limited and or contradictory.

Recent evidence also suggests that BCAA-stimulated muscle protein synthesis is also limited in duration. A recent review on the role of BCAAs in stimulating protein synthesis following exercise stated:

" Providing increased exogenous BCAAs is likely to stimulate MPS (and possibly decreased muscle protein breakdown), but the effect is likely to be short-lived given the muscle–full phenomenon."

What about real world athletic performance?

Within the context of a high protein diet, extra BCAAs don't appear to be particularly effective. I don't know of anyone that added extra LBM because they started supplementing with BCAAs. There are some who feel they're helpful for helping to maintain LBM during a cutting phase. This is something that has not been directly evaluated under controlled conditions, so it's strictly speculative at this point, but it would stand to reason that BCAA use during reduced calorie intakes may help preserve lean body mass.

Will Brink's Recommendation

Although BCAAs supplementation may or may not be effective, it's expensive when one factors in the amounts needed to boost performance. The good news, however, is that proteins, in particular whey protein, are very high in BCAAs and this may be yet another reason whey is so popular with athletes and so impressive in the research.

In relationship to the functions they play in the body, branched chain amino acids get a thumbs up from me, but as a supplement they get a thumbs down, at this time. It's far more cost effective to use a high BCAA content protein supplement than to take BCAAs supplements in capsule form, due to the high doses needed.

References

Davis JM, Welsh RS, De Volve KL, Alderson NA. Effects of branched–chain amino acids and carbohydrate on fatigue during intermittent, high–intensity running. Int J Sports Med. 1999 Jul;20(5):309-14.

Kreider, RB, Miriel V and Bertun E. Amino acid supplementation and exercise performance. Analysis of the proposed ergogenic value. Sports Med. 1993 Sep;16(3):190-209.

Mero A. Leucine supplementation and intensive training. Sports Med. 1999 Jun;27(6):347-58.

Mittleman, KD, Ricci MR and Bailey SP. Branched–chain amino acids prolong exercise during heat stress in men and women. Med Sci Sports Exerc. 1998 Jan;30(1):83-91.

Rennie MJ, Bohe J, Smith K, Wackerhage H, Greenhaff P. Branched–chain amino acids as fuels and anabolic signals in human muscle. J Nutr. 2006 Jan;136 (1 Suppl):264S-8S.

Wagenmakers, AJ. Amino acid supplements to improve athletic performance. Curr Opin Clin Nutr Metab Care. 1999 Nov;2(6):539-44.

Williams, MH. Facts and fallacies of purported ergogenic amino acid supplements. Clin Sports Med. 1999 Jul;18(3):633-49.

☙

CITRULLINE

What is it?

Citrulline is a non-essential amino acid that plays a role in a variety of metabolic processes. Citrulline is an essential player in the detoxification on ammonia and other byproducts of metabolism, such as lactate. Citrulline readily converts to the amino acid arginine and is an intermediate in the urea cycle.

What is it supposed to do?

Citrulline is reported to improve performance by improving the clearance of ammonia and lactate, both of which build up quickly during exercise and cause a decrease in performance as levels increase. Citrulline is claimed to improve aerobic capacity and endurance by influencing lactic acid metabolism—ultimately reducing fatigue. As most people know, ammonia is toxic to cells. The body deals with ammonia via what is called the urea cycle, by which potentially toxic metabolites are made less toxic and excreted via the kidneys and urine. As a part of the urea cycle, citrulline is essential to detoxify and remove ammonia as well as lactate.

As mentioned, citrulline readily converts to arginine, which has gotten much attention recently due to it's being a precursor to nitric oxide (NO), a key signaling molecule (see arginine section for additional comments on NO) in the human body. NO is a vasodilator that mediates the relaxation of smooth muscle. NO is a key signaling molecule in the human body for a huge number of functions and is beyond the scope of this chapter. In summary: Citrulline may improve performance by improving the clearance of ammonia and lactate during exercise, but other effects may include an improvement in ATP replenishment post-workout.

What does the research have to say?

Clinically, citrulline has shown promise in the treatment of various human afflictions, such as fatigue in geriatric settings as well as improvements in mental acuity and resistance to mental fatigue and improvements in reducing fatigue in postoperative patients. Citrulline has been used in various European countries for almost two decades. Though human studies are limited, they do exist, and findings have been promising (with some exceptions). Animal studies find improvements in endurance as well reductions in ammonia in response to intense exercise. One recent study done with eighteen men complaining of fatigue (but with no documented disease) were studied. According to the study:

" CM ingestion resulted in a significant reduction in the sensation of fatigue, a 34% increase in the rate of oxidative ATP production during exercise, and a 20% increase in the rate of phosphocreatine recovery after exercise... "

This result led the researchers to conclude:

"...the changes in muscle metabolism produced by CM treatment indicate that CM may promote aerobic energy production. "

Other studies, although limited, generally support the use of citrulline as a supplement that improves endurance, but effects on strength and or LBM are not well studied. All is not perfect however as a recent study actually found citrulline reduced time to exhaustion in, healthy male and female volunteers given citrulline compared to placebo. Translated, in this study, citrulline actually decreased endurance! The study also found the group given citrulline had higher rates of perceived exertion during exercise. The study concluded:

"...contrary to the hypothesized improvement in treadmill time following L–citrulline ingestion, there is a reduction in treadmill time following L–citrulline ingestion... "

What about real world athletic performance?

Very little feedback has come in with this supplement, as it's fairly new to the sport nutrition market and not well known. Endurance athletes have generally been positive about it and, as expected, strength athletes have been negative. Admittedly, the sample size was small.

Will Brink's Recommendation

As most people know, "hemodialator" supplements are simply based on arginine. Citrulline appears to be better at increasing both arginine and NO then arginine itself. So, those taking arginine–based hemodialators might be better off taking citrulline. The minimum dose for effects appears to be 6 grams, taken before workouts on an empty stomach. Higher doses (up to 18 g) have been used in studies without any apparent ill effects.

Although citrulline will probably have no direct effects on strength and LBM, it may still benefit strength athletes indirectly by allowing a few more reps (due to its effects on lactate and ammonia) with a given weight and perhaps, improved aerobic metabolism, cellular energy production, and muscular recovery. I am going to put citrulline in the "might be worth a try" category and a borderline thumbs up at this time.

References

Bendahan D, Mattei JP, Ghattas B, et al. Citrulline/malate promotes aerobic energy production in human exercising muscle. Br J Sports Med. 2002 Aug;36(4):282-9.

Callis A, Magnan de Bornier B, Serrano JJ, et al. Activity of citrulline malate on acid–base balance and blood ammonia and amino acid levels. Study in the animal and in man. Arzneimittelforschung. 1991 Jun;41(6):660-3.

Hickner RC, Tanner CJ, Evans CA, et al. L–citrulline reduces time to exhaustion and insulin response to a graded exercise test. Med Sci Sports Exerc. 2006 Apr;38(4):660-6.

Janeira MA, Maia JR, Santos PJ. Citrulline malate effects on the aerobic–anaerobic threshold and in post-exercise blood lactate recovery. Med Sci Sports Exerc. 1998 30(5), Supplement abstract 880.

Meneguello MO, Mendonca JR, Lancha AH Jr, Costa Rosa LF. Effect of arginine, ornithine and citrulline supplementation upon performance and metabolism of trained rats. Cell Biochem Funct. 2003 Mar;21(1):85-91.

Wilkerson JE, Batterson DL, Horvath SM. Exercise induced changes in blood ammonia levels in humans. Eur J Appl Physiol 1977;37:255-263.

ф

L–GLUTAMINE

What is it?

L–glutamine is a conditionally essential amino acid. It's considered to be one of the most important amino acids when the body is under severe stress, such as following surgery, trauma, burns, etc.

What is it supposed to do?

Glutamine participates in a wide variety of non-protein activities in the body. Supplemental glutamine may enhance immunity and promote muscle recovery, along with other potential health benefits.

What does the research say for athletic performance?

The 'non-essential' amino acid glutamine has been getting a great deal of attention over the past few years in sport nutrition publications and scientific journals and for good reason. Though it might not be considered "essential," glutamine appears to have many potential benefits for people interested in gaining new muscle and/or preserving that hard earned muscle. Glutamine is required for countless functions in the human body from immune system function, to liver function, to gastrointestinal integrity, to name only a few. Supplement companies have taken to adding glutamine to various products and athletes have taken to adding glutamine to their diet.

For example, it is well known that low plasma glutamine levels are associated with a loss of lean body mass (muscle) and intense exercise is known to reduce glutamine stores. One study attempted to directly link glutamine levels with lean tissue loss.

The study divided 34 healthy men into three groups. One group did intense aerobic work (running), another group did intense anaerobic work (weight lifting and sprinting), and the third group was sedentary (aka couch potatoes).

The authors of this study found that the greatest loss of muscle was found in those men who had the lowest baseline glutamine levels, which demonstrates just how important this amino acid is for maintaining hard earned muscle tissue. Plain and simple, the harder you train the more glutamine you drain! Because of its potential effects on the immune system, the use of glutamine may also help to prevent overtraining syndrome (OTS) in athletes who train too long and too hard. Several studies have suggested glutamine levels may be indicators for OTS.

Another interesting effect of glutamine is it may increase growth hormone levels (GH). One study took nine healthy subjects and fed them two grams (2000 mg) of glutamine dissolved in a cola drink. Eight out of the nine subjects responded to the oral glutamine intake with a four-fold increase in growth hormone (GH) output.

This study was particularly interesting because: a) the glutamine was given orally and not intravenously, as in other studies; and b) the study only used two grams of glutamine. Most studies that showed any effect on GH used very large doses and were given directly into the veins of the poor participants.

That only two grams of glutamine taken orally had such an effect of GH bodes well for the use of glutamine by athletes. Whether or not a short spike in GH will lead to new muscle is another question however, and in truth, short-lived spikes in GH in healthy young athletes do not appear to affect muscle mass.

Finally, glutamine may be useful in replenishing glycogen stores in muscle after intense exercise. Glycogen is stored in muscle cells for energy and other functions such as cell volume. As most athletes know, glycogen is rather important stuff to have around when you want to perform well. The researchers took six healthy volunteers and made them exercise at 70-140% of maximal oxygen consumption to deplete their muscle glycogen stores. They found that the glutamine enhanced glycogen storage after the intense bout of exercise. Exactly how glutamine improves glycogen storage is not clear.

It might somehow improve the uptake of glucose into muscle directly, or it might be that the glutamine is itself being converted into glucose and then being stored as glycogen in the muscles. The authors of the study seem to suggests the latter. Either way, this might just be one more amazing benefit of this amino acid for athletes.

What about real world athletic performance?

Many trainers recommend glutamine supplementation as a preventive measure, to limit the depletion of muscle glutamine stores that occur during strenuous exercise. Needless to state, no one have ever exploded with muscle from the simple addition of glutamine to the diet.

Will Brink's Recommendation

Although it doesn't directly enhance performance or LBM, glutamine gets a thumbs up as a general health improving supplement that appears to have applications for athletes. 5-20 grams per day of glutamine added to a post-workout shake is the norm. Don't expect any changes in LBM or performance from this supplement regardless of the hype marketing you will see on L-glutamine, but there may be secondary benefits to athletes.

References

Phillips GC. Glutamine: the nonessential amino acid for performance enhancement. Curr Sports Med Rep 2007 Jul;6(4):265-8.

Keast D, Arstein D, Harper W, Fry RW, et al. Depression of plasma glutamine concentration after exercise stress and its possible influence on the immune system. Med J Aust. 1995 Jan 2;162(1):15-8.

Newsholme EA. Biochemical mechanisms to explain immunosuppression in well trained and over trained athletes. Int J Sports Med. 1994 Oct;15 Suppl 3:S142-7.

Varnier, M. and G. P. Leese, et al. Stimulatory effect of glutamine on glycogen accumulation in human skeletal muscle. Am J. Physiol. Aug;269(2 Pt 1):E309-15.

Welbourne TC. Increased plasma bicarbonate and growth hormone after an oral glutamine load. Am J Clin Nutr. 1995 May;61(5):1058-61.

φ

ORNITHINE ALPHA–KETOGLUTARATE (OKG)

What is it?

Ornithine is a non-protein amino acid that is an integral part of the urea cycle,which the body uses to dispose of excess nitrogen. Ornithine alpha–ketoglutarate is a salt of ornithine and alpha–ketoglutarate, which is the carbon skeleton of the amino acid glutamate.

What is it supposed to do?

Ornithine alpha–ketoglutarate is alleged to have anti-catabolic/anabolic and immune modulating activities. It is also used to increase the secretion of growth hormone.

What does the research say for athletic performance?

There's extensive research on the value of supplementing enteral/parenteral feedings of burn/trauma patients with ornithine alpha–ketoglutarate. Experiments with both rodents and humans have demonstrated that OKG limits muscle protein breakdown, improves gut health and increases the muscle glutamine pool.

OKG also has immunomodulating effects: in rats, OKG supplementation increases the weight of the thymus (an important organ in the immune system) and improves the responses of specific immune cell types (macrophages and neutrophils) in under burn or stress conditions.

OKG also stimulates the secretion of important anabolic hormones. Fifteen grams of OKG added to the feeding solutions of children receiving total parenteral nutrition resulted in improved growth and a significant increase in IGF–1. Enterally fed trauma patients also experienced increased levels of IGF–1, along with insulin and growth hormone vs. controls.

At least part of OKG's effects are mediated by its role as an arginine precursor and the latter's function as a substrate for nitric oxide (NO) synthesis. It's clear that OKG is a far more potent precursor for arginine synthesis than ornithine itself.

Data also suggests OKG may be of benefit to aging populations with age related loss of muscle mass (sarcopenia).

What does all this mean for healthy athletes?

There is virtually no useful data on the utility of OKG supplementation in healthy humans. Rat studies are mildly suggestive of some potential benefits, such as enhanced insulin secretion, which might be useful for pre- and/or post-workout recovery. A study on rats exercised to exhaustion demonstrated that OKG increased glutamine synthesis and resulted in enhanced buffering of ammonia. This is an effect that—if it occurs in humans—might enhance performance or recovery.

OKG is sometimes added to NO supplements, thanks to its role in NO production. Since OKG converts to arginine, however, and NO supps already contain arginine (usually as AAKG), its presence is redundant. OKG supplementation appears to increase locomotor activity in rats, which means it may have a stimulating effect and could provide a workout boost, but it's unknown if it has this effect in humans. Many NO supplements contain caffeine or other stimulants, which makes it impossible to tell what—if any— stimulating effects OKG itself might have.

As for its effects on GH, there is no evidence that the temporary spikes in GH induced by amino acids have any effect on mass gains or strength, as outlined in the section on GH releasing supplements.

What about real world athletic performance?

Some give high marks to NO supplements as workout energizers, apart from the "pump," so it's possible – but far from certain—that OKG (if included in the formula) could contribute to that effect. As far as OKG alone, feedback from people taking it alone is essentially non-existent. Very few people consume OKG alone, or in doses that reflect what's used in studies, so it's virtually impossible to get accurate feedback on OKG.

Will Brink's Recommendation

My recommendations for OKG are essentially the same as for arginine; it may have some health uses, but I see no reason to recommend it to anyone looking to add mass or strength at this time. Although useful human data is lacking on OKG's effects on strength or LBM, what is known, however, is that NO and GH supps do nada (read jack sh&%) for gains in lean body mass, so whatever positive effects OKG may have, muscle growth isn't one of them. It does appear to have some medical uses, and perhaps health uses, but it gets thumbs down as a muscle builder or performance enhancer at this time.

References

Walrand S. Ornithine alpha–ketoglutarate: could it be a new therapeutic option for sarcopenia? J Nutr Health Aging. 2010 Aug;14(7):570-7.

Chromiak JA, Antonio J. Use of amino acids as growth hormone–releasing agents by athletes. Nutrition. 2002 Jul–Aug;18(7–8):657-61.

Cynober L. Ornithine alpha–ketoglutarate as a potent precursor of arginine and nitric oxide: a new job for an old friend. J Nutr. 2004 Oct;134(10 Suppl):2858S-2862S.

Cynober LA. The use of alpha–ketoglutarate salts in clinical nutrition and metabolic care. Curr Opin Clin Nutr Metab Care. 1999 Jan;2(1):33-7.

Jeevanandam M, Petersen SR. Substrate fuel kinetics in enterally fed trauma patients supplemented with ornithine alpha ketoglutarate. Clin Nutr. 1999 Aug;18(4):209-17.

Le Boucher J, Eurengbiol, Farges MC, et al. Modulation of immune response with ornithine A–ketoglutarate in burn injury: an arginine or glutamine dependency? Nutrition. 1999 Oct;15(10):773-7.

Le Bricon T, Cynober L, Baracos VE. Ornithine alpha–ketoglutarate limits muscle protein breakdown without stimulating tumor growth in rats bearing Yoshida ascites hepatoma. Metabolism. 1994 Jul;43(7):899-905.

Meneguello MO, Mendonca JR, Lancha AH, et al. Effect of arginine, ornithine and citrulline supplementation upon performance and metabolism of trained rats. Cell Biochem Funct. 2003 Mar;21(1):85-91.

Moinard C, Dauge V, Cynober L. Ornithine alpha–ketoglutarate supplementation influences motor activity in healthy rats. Clin Nutr. 2004 Aug;23(4):485-90.

Moinard C, Caldefie F, Walrand S, et al. Effects of ornithine 2–oxoglutarate on neutrophils in stressed rats: evidence for the involvement of nitric oxide and polyamines. Clin Sci (Lond). 2002 Mar;102(3):287-95.

Moinard C, Caldefie F, Walrand S, et al. Involvement of glutamine, arginine, and polyamines in the action of ornithine alpha–ketoglutarate on macrophage functions in stressed rats. J Leukoc Biol. 2000 Jun;67(6):834-40.

Moinard C, Chauveau B, Walrand S, et al. Phagocyte functions in stressed rats: comparison of modulation by glutamine, arginine and ornithine 2–oxoglutarate. Clin Sci (Lond). 1999 Jul;97(1):59-65.

Moukarzel AA, Goulet O, Salas JS, et al. Growth retardation in children receiving long–term total parenteral nutrition: effects of ornithine alpha–ketoglutarate. Am J Clin Nutr. 1994 Sep;60(3):408-13.

Robinson LE, Bussiere FI, Le Boucher J, et al. Amino acid nutrition and immune function in tumour–bearing rats: a comparison of glutamine–, arginine–and ornithine 2–oxoglutarate–supplemented diets. Clin Sci (Lond). 1999 Dec;97(6):657-69.

Schneid C, De Bandt JP, Cynober L, et al. In vivo induction of insulin secretion by ornithine alpha–ketoglutarate: involvement of nitric oxide and glutamine. Metabolism. 2003 Mar;52(3):344-50.

Vaubourdolle M, Coudray–Lucas C, Jardel A, et al. Action of enterally administered ornithine alpha–ketoglutarate on protein breakdown in skeletal muscle and liver of the burned rat. JPEN J Parenter Enteral Nutr. 1991 Sep-Oct;15(5):517-20.

Φ

TAURINE

What is it?

Taurine is a ubiquitous non-essential amino acid found throughout the human body, similar to glutamine. It's considered non-essential because the body can make taurine from the amino acids methionine and cysteine, with the help of vitamin B6.

Although it may be non-essential, supplemental taurine may have some potentially interesting effects from which athletes may benefit. In fact, it should probably be listed as conditionally essential, which means under certain circumstances, it becomes essential to the human body.

What is it supposed to do?

Much of taurine's exact role in human biology is still being elucidated, but what has been looked at is compelling. Taurine is intimately connected with cell volume, blood pressure, insulin metabolism, the ability of muscles to contract correctly and hundreds of other functions known and yet unknown.

What does the research say for athletic performance?

For example, there is a steady decline in taurine levels as we age, which may lead to a host of problems. One study in which rats were fed taurine at 1.5 percent of calories found taurine supplementation blunted age related declines in serum IGF–1, an important anabolic hormone essential to muscle growth and protein synthesis.

Another study found that supplemental taurine in aging rats corrected the age related decline in the ability of the rat's muscle to contract. The study suggested that an age related decline of taurine content could play a role in the alteration of electrical and contractile properties of muscles observed during aging and that supplemental taurine corrected the decline. The study concluded:

"...these findings may indicate a potential application of taurine in ensuring normal muscle function in the elderly."

This has very exciting possibilities in aging populations, but human trials are still lacking. Another exciting area of research for taurine is its possible role in managing diabetes and improving insulin sensitivity. Several studies in both rats and humans suggest taurine can play a role in improving several indices of diabetes, such as insulin metabolism, high cholesterol levels and high blood pressure, as well as others. Diabetics appear to be chronically low in taurine.

For example, one study found taurine attenuated hypertension and improved insulin sensitivity in rats made insulin resistant by a high fructose diet. Treatment with 2 percent taurine put in the rats' drinking water prevented the blood pressure elevation and attenuated the hyperinsulinemia (high insulin levels) in fructose fed rats and prevented the large spike in glucose levels in response to an oral glucose load.

The study concluded:

"...thus, taurine supplementation could be beneficial in circumventing metabolic alterations in insulin resistance."

Several studies have found this effect in rats fed taurine and made diabetic. One human study looked at the ability of taurine to prevent blood platelet aggregation or "sticky" blood cells in diabetics. This is important because "sticky" blood platelets are related to the development of heart attacks and is a particular issue to diabetics. The study found that supplemental taurine made the diabetic's blood aggregation or "stickiness" equal to that of healthy controls.

What about real world athletic performance?

So what use does taurine have to athletes and healthy people? Well again, as is so often the case, human studies in healthy athletes are lacking, so it's difficult or near impossible to make solid recommendations at this time. Taurine might be a great supplement to healthy athletes or it may only work in those populations who chronically lack taurine in their tissues, such as the aging, diabetics and others.

One thing is for sure, as with pretty much all amino acids, multi-gram doses will probably be needed for any effect and any product that sprinkles in a few milligrams will be of little use to the buyer.

Will Brink's Recommendation

It would be great if we had solid data showing some positive effects in athletes. And it would be nice if we knew what the effective dose was. Sadly, we have neither at this time. However, due to the sheer amount of overall data we have, I am still giving taurine a tentative thumbs up as a "worth a try" supplement.

References

Anuradha CV, Balakrishnan SD. Taurine attenuates hypertension and improves insulin sensitivity in the fructose–fed rat, an animal model of insulin resistance. Can J Physiol Pharmacol. 1999 Oct;77(10):749-54.

Dawson R Jr, Liu S, Eppler B, Patterson T. Effects of dietary taurine supplementation or deprivation in aged male Fischer 344 rats. Mech Ageing Dev. 1999 Feb 1;107(1):73-91.

Franconi F, Bennardini F, Mattana A, et al. Plasma and platelet taurine are reduced in subjects with insulin–dependent diabetes mellitus: effects of taurine supplementation. Am J Clin Nutr. 1995 May;61(5):1115-9.

Hansen, SH. The role of taurine in diabetes and the development of diabetic complications. Diabetes Metab Res Rev. 2001 Sep–Oct;17(5):330-46.

Nakaya Y, Minami A, Harada N, et al. Taurine improves insulin sensitivity in the Otsuka Long-Evans Tokushima Fatty rat, a model of spontaneous type 2 diabetes. Am J Clin Nutr. 2000 Jan;71(1):54-8.

ф

L–TYROSINE

What is it?

One amino acid that has not gotten a great deal of attention by athletes is the amino acid L–tyrosine. L–tyrosine is found in high amounts in protein foods and the body can make L–tyrosine from amino acid phenylalanine, technically making it a "non-essential" amino acid.

What is it supposed to do?

This often overlooked amino acid plays many important roles in human metabolism. L–tyrosine is a precursor or "building block" to the neurotransmitters responsible for maintaining metabolic rate. L–tyrosine is the direct precursor to stimulatory neurotransmitters such as epinephrine and norepinephrine (i.e. adrenaline) as well as certain thyroid hormones and dopamine.

Due to the fact that tyrosine is essential to the production of all the above stimulatory hormones and neurotransmitters, some consider it an amino acid with mild stimulant-like properties to the metabolism and mental focus. Some weight loss supplements contain L–tyrosine in an attempt to supply this essential building block in hopes it will help maintain a higher metabolism.

What does the research say for athletic performance?

Though tyrosine has not been shown to be an effective weight loss agent on its own, several studies have shown it can improve the anorectic (appetite suppressive) effects of the herbal weight loss products containing ephedrine and caffeine and OTC diet drugs containing phenylpropanolamine.

Several studies done by the US Army showed soldiers given supplemental L–tyrosine were more resistant to cold temperatures than those not getting the amino acid. One recent study found that

21 cadets, fed 2 grams of tyrosine a day then subjected to a demanding military combat training course, reduced the effects of stress and fatigue on cognitive task performance. So, tyrosine may be a stress fighting nutrient.

What about real world athletic performance?

It's not uncommon that people are given advice on what to eat in regards to the food's amino acid content. For example, many people have probably heard at one time or another, "If you want to be more alert, eat a high protein food." This advice is probably due to the high L–tyrosine content of the food. Conversely, people are also given advice that to relax, they should eat foods such as milk and turkey, which are high in the amino acid L–tryptophan. L–tryptophan is a building block of the neurotransmitter serotonin, which is known to help with sleep and relaxation.

Some strength athletes have found that by taking 500 to 2000 mg of tyrosine prior to exercise, they have more energy, but no studies to date have found this to be an effect of tyrosine.

However, because it may be a mild stimulant and works at the level of the central nervous system, people using MAO inhibitors, pregnant women, people with high blood pressure and people sensitive to stimulants, should probably avoid high doses of tyrosine.

Will Brink's Recommendation

For general mental focus and stress fighting, as well as for pre-workout, or mixed with the various weight loss agents, tyrosine gets a thumbs up; but for any direct effects on anabolism (muscle growth) it gets a thumbs down. It tends to work quite well with caffeine in my experience.

References

Deijen J.B., Wientjes C.J., Vullinghs H.F., et al. Tyrosine improves cognitive performance and reduces blood pressure in cadets after one week of a combat training course. Brain Res Bull. 1999 Jan 15;48(2):203-9.

Hull, K. M. and Maher T. J. Effects of L–tyrosine on mixed–acting sympathomimetic–induced pressor actions. Pharmacol Biochem Behav. 43/4 (1992), p. 1047-52.

Hull, K. M. and Maher T. J. L–tyrosine potentiates the anorexia induced by mixed–acting sympathomimetic drugs in hyperphagic rats. Pharmacol Exp Ther. 255/2 (1990), p. 403-9.

Owasoyo J.O., Neri D.F., Lamberth J.G. Tyrosine and its potential use as a countermeasure to performance decrement in military sustained operations. Aviat Space Environ Med. 1992 May;63(5):364-9.

Salter C.A. Dietary tyrosine as an aid to stress resistance among troops. Mil Med. 1989 Mar;154(3):144-6.

ቀ

Chapter 2

METABOLITES

There are a number of naturally occurring metabolites that can be taken in supplemental form, to raise levels in the body higher than can be achieved through diet alone. The idea is to amplify the effects that the compound has, with the goal of enhancing performance and/or improving body composition.

Because they are compounds naturally produced in the body, toxicity is less likely to be a problem, although there may be side effects from ingesting excessive amounts. The compounds that follow aren't an exhaustive list: there are hundreds of potentially useful metabolites that might be taken in supplemental form. These are simply the ones that most commonly turn up in commercial supplements.

It's a list that will almost certainly be added to in the future. It's important to remember that a compound that's ineffective for

Metabolites Covered

- ❖ Agmatine
- ❖ Arachidonic Acid
- ❖ Creatine Monohydrate
- ❖ Carnitine
- ❖ DHEA
- ❖ 7–Keto DHEA
- ❖ GABA
- ❖ HMB and KIC
- ❖ Phosphatidylserine
- ❖ Ribose

building muscle or increasing strength might still have positive effects on health and/or prevention of disease. Your state of health will have a significant impact on your results, so certain nutrients might be worthwhile to take, in spite of having little direct effect on LBM or performance.

AGMATINE

What is it?

Agmatine is essentially a decarboxylated form of the amino acid arginine. Agmatine is an intermediate in polyamine biosynthesis and is produced in the body enzymatically via the decarboxylation of arginine by arginine decarboxylase.

It can be considered a downstream metabolite of arginine and is often referred to as a "bioactive metabolite" of arginine. Agmatine is found in different areas of the body in varying concentrations, with agmatine being found the stomach, the heart, small intestine, spleen, adrenal glands, skeletal muscle, and of course the brain. Agmatine will most likely be found in other areas of the body also.

What is it supposed to do?

Agmatine appears to play an extensive role in the human body, some which is still being elucidated. The various pathways and potential effects of agmatine in various systems is extensive and extremely complicated, so I will need to keep it narrowed down as best I can to the areas of interest/concern to athletic endeavors, which is the main concern of this book.

Agmatine appears to act as a neurotransmitter in the brain and plays some role in Insulin metabolism as well as having direct effects on the release of some peptide hormones (GH, IGF–1, LH, LHRH, etc) as well as non-peptide hormones (e.g., testosterone). Its exact role in the release and or metabolism of these hormones is poorly understood in humans.

Other claims for agmatine are as a possible memory enhancer, antidepressant, and modulator of nitric oxide (NO). It's also claimed to potentially aid post-workout recovery. Finally, agmatine is noted as a possible pain modulator which might help athletes control pain due to injuries and such. Most applicable to athletes, due to its possible effects on various hormones, it's being claimed it will increase endurance/enhance performance and decrease body fat.

However, the major thrust of the advertising and marketing claims is as a supplement that can enhance the "pump" one gets in the gym similar to the claims being made about arginine-based products (e.g., NO2 and the ilk) and citrulline products. See arginine and or citrulline sections of this book for more additional information on that issue.

What does the research say for athletic performance?

This is where things get real fuzzy as it applies to the above claims that are supposed to benefit athletes. The research that exists is mostly in vitro (test tube) or animal (rats, to be more specific), and most of it has no real application to athletes, at least not directly. Actual research looking at endpoints of interest to athletes, such as effects on strength, body composition, endurance, or performance in general simply don't exist at this time.

In rats, fairly large doses of agmatine administered intracerebroventricularly directly into their brains) rapidly increased the release of luteinizing hormone (LH) in a dose-related fashion in "ovariectomized, ovarian steroid primed rats."

If you're an ovariectomized ovarian steroid primed rat, my apologies, but I think that will leave out most of the readers of this book!

Probably the most promising—and best supported—use for agmatine is as a pain modulator. Interestingly, it's also found to greatly reduce withdrawal symptoms from morphine as well as augment the effects of morphine on pain—at least in rats.

For example, one study found exposing rats to morphine for seven days resulted in marked withdrawal symptoms (as expected) but agmatine treatment along with morphine significantly decreasing the withdrawal symptoms and augmented the effects of morphine on pain. As the authors of another study concluded;

" We conclude that agmatine, an endogenous substance derived from arginine, can modulate both acute and chronic pain."

It should be noted that most of the research done on rats is done as either injections or other routes that bypassed digestion, so the oral use of agmatine is an additional question mark.

An interesting side note regarding the research: pharmaceutical companies have been looking at "agmatine analogs" as possible GH–releasing agents which may have applications to athletes and aging populations in the future, but again, little definitive data exists.

What about real world athletic performance?

Because agmatine is so new to the market as a supplement there is limited feedback. The feedback that does exist has been mixed, with some people reporting similar "improved pumps in the gym" similar to the NO products. Some report no effects at all however.

Will Brink's Recommendation

To say recommending agmatine as a supplement to human beings is premature is an understatement. To say it's premature to recommend it to athletes as a supplement in hopes of seeing improvements in body comp or performance is the mother of all understatements. Agmatine is a very interesting and possibly promising supplement, but the unknowns exceed what we know about this compound by a factor of a zillion.

As it also appears to play a role in so many systems in the body, the number of people who should avoid this supplement due to some medical condition or possible negative drug interaction will be quite large. It could have interactions (positive or negative) with various antidepressant medications, blood pressure medications, various heart medications, various pain medications, and many others, some of which are not even known at this time.

Agmatine gets a firm thumbs down from me and is not recommended at this time.

References

Abe K, Abe Y, and Saito H. Agmatine suppresses nitric oxide production in microglia. Brain Res. 872: 141-148, 2000.

Agmatine and Imidazolines: Their Novel Receptors and Enzymes Volume 1009 published December 2003. Ann. N.Y. Acad. Sci. 1009: 106–115 (2003).

Aricioglu F, Means A, Regunathan S. Effect of agmatine on the development of morphine dependence in rats: potential role of cAMP system. Eur J Pharmacol. 2004 Nov 19;504(3):191-7.

Aricioglu–Kartal F, Regunathan S. Effect of chronic morphine treatment on the biosynthesis of agmatine in rat brain and other tissues. Life Sci. 71:1695-1701, 2002.

Aricioglu–Kartal F, Regunathan S. Effect of chronic morphine treatment on the biosynthesis of agmatine in rat brain and other tissues. Life Sci. 2002 Aug 23;71(14):1695-701.

Gao, Y, et al. Agmatine: a novel vasodilator substance. Life Sci. 57(8): PL83-86, 1995.

Kalra SP, Pearson E, Sahu A, Kalra PS. Agmatine, a novel hypothalamic amine, stimulates pituitary luteinizing hormone release in vivo and hypothalamic luteinizing hormone–releasing hormone release in vitro. Neurosci Lett. 1995 Jul 21;194(3):165-8.

Li YF, et al. Antidepressant–like effect of agmatine and its possible mechanism. Eur J Pharmacol. 2003 May 23;469(1-3):81-8.

Morgan NG, Chan SL, Brown CA, Tsoli E. Characterization of the imidazoline binding site involved in regulation of insulin secretion. Ann N Y Acad Sci. 1995 Jul 12;763:361-73.

Raasch W, Regunathan S, Li G, Reis DJ. Agmatine, the bacterial amine, is widely distributed in mammalian tissues. Life Sci. 1995;56(26):2319-30.

Raghavan SA, Dikshit M. Vascular regulation by the L–arginine metabolites, nitric oxide and agmatine. Pharmacol Res. 49(5):397-414. Review, 2004.

Reis DJ, Regunathan S. Is agmatine a novel neurotransmitter in brain? Trends Pharmacol Sci. 2000 May;21(5):187-93.

Reis DJ, Regunathan S. Agmatine: a novel neurotransmitter? Adv Pharmacol. 1998;42:645-9.

Stewart LS, McKay BE. Acquisition deficit and time-dependent retrograde amnesia for contextual fear conditioning in agmatine-treated rats. Behav Pharmacol. 2000 Feb;11(1):93-7.

Yananli H, Goren MZ, Berkman K, Aricioglu F. Effect of agmatine on brain l–citrulline production during morphine withdrawal in rats: A microdialysis study in nucleus accumbens. Brain Res. 2007 Feb 9;1132(1):51-58, 2006.

Zarandi M, Serfozo P, Zsigo J, Deutch AH, et al. Potent agonists of growth hormone–releasing hormone. II. Pept Res. 5(4):190-3, 1992.

ቀ

ARACHIDONIC ACID

What is it?

Arachidonic acid (AA) is a naturally occurring polyunsaturated fat, belonging to the omega–6 family of fatty acids and is found in cell membrane phospholipids. It's formed in the human body from the essential fatty acid linoleic acid (LA) or ingested preformed in various foods, with highest amounts found in red meat, egg yolks, and other animals based foods. From AA, highly unsaturated biologically active compounds such as prostaglandins, prostacyclin (PGI12), leukotrienes, and thromboxanes are formed.

What is it supposed to do?

The metabolism of AA is extremely complicated and far beyond the scope of this section. The many biologically active downstream metabolites of AA mentioned above are still under investigation, with new roles for each being discovered all the time. Relating to the issue that concerns the reader (e.g., effects on strength, performance, and body composition), AA plays a role in the inflammatory response, which appears to have direct effects on protein synthesis. In particular, the prostaglandin PGF2a has been identified as an important mediator of protein synthesis. In theory, an increase in the tissue levels of PGF2a (via ingestion of AA) might alter the anabolic to catabolic balance which would increase muscle mass.

Other lines of evidence that support AA metabolites as being essential for protein synthesis come from studies that found that the cyclooxygenase (COX) enzyme inhibitors ibuprofen and acetaminophen greatly diminish the anabolic response to resistance exercise by inhibiting the normal post-exercise increase in levels of PGF2a. As these OTC drugs exhibit their anti-inflammatory actions by inhibiting the synthesis of prostaglandins, and it's been found they reduce protein synthetic rates in response to weight training, it's additional support for the concept that prostaglandins play an essential role in the anabolic response to exercise. Again, that's a generalization of an extremely complicated system. The essential take home of the above is, prostaglandins are derived from dietary and in vivo conversion of AA and appear up-regulate recovery mechanisms including: inflammation and protein synthesis within skeletal muscle in response to resistance training.

What does the research have to say?

Most of the research that suggests AA has anabolic and or anti-catabolic effects via its conversion to PGF2a (and perhaps other metabolites yet to be elucidated) has been in vitro (test tube) research. Other than intellectually interesting, very little can be concluded as it applies to living systems. Although there have been studies that examined the effects of humans ingesting AA, these studies did not examine the effects on whole body protein synthesis or skeletal muscle mass or tissue levels of PGF2a. However, one recent study did look directly at the effects of AA on strength and body composition.

The 50 day study consisted of thirty-one resistance trained males who were randomly assigned to a placebo (P: n = 16; 1 g capsulated corn oil/day) or AA group (AA: n = 15; 1 g capsulated AA/day). Although diet was not controlled for (a major flaw of this study, BTW), they were given supplemental protein powder to assure an adequate protein intake while participating in a 4 day per week resistance training regimen which consisted of a twice per week upper/lower split.

The researchers examined various downstream metabolites of AA, such as: prostaglandin E2 (PGE2), prostaglandin F2α (PGF2α), interleukin–6 (IL–6), as well as hormonal effects on free testosterone, total testosterone and cortisol. They also took muscle biopsies to look at any changes in myosin heavy chain isoform. The study did not find statistically significant differences between the group getting the AA and the placebo group. There was a trend in the changes of some of the outcomes examined, but none of them reached statistical significance which equates to no differences between groups.

The researchers concluded:

" Results suggest that AA supplementation during resistance training may exert some potentially favorable alterations IL–6 levels and prostaglandin levels and that additional research is necessary to further examine this hypothesis."

What about real world athletic performance?

Interestingly, feedback for this supplement has been generally positive, though not universally so. Some people claim they get stronger and feel additionally sore from their workouts, which they attribute to the known effects of AA on inflammation.

Will Brink's Recommendation

The use of AA as a dietary supplement is a controversial and contentious idea. The reason is that AA is associated with a long list of possible diseases and inflammatory conditions due to its role as a precursor to the pro-inflammatory metabolites mentioned above. Inflammation, and a high intake of AA or LA (linoleic acid: omega–6 lipid), is associated with all manner of inflammatory conditions and or diseases that are known to have chronic inflammation as an important mediator of the process. It's generally believed that the high intakes of LA and low intakes of omega–3 fats (which have anti-inflammatory effects) are partially responsible for the high levels of various inflammatory conditions suffered by typically affluent Western countries.

The list of conditions and diseases either caused by or negatively impacted by, inflammation is huge, but includes: coronary heart disease (CHD), psoriasis, asthma and rheumatoid arthritis, diabetes, and many other conditions and diseases.

Of course inflammation is not all bad and we would not live long without an inflammatory response to various pathogens and other challenges where the inflammatory response is an essential part of our immune system. The issue is chronically elevated inflammation. Again, this is a huge topic, an incredibly complicated topic, and to make matters worse, a topic with plenty of unknowns.

Thus, no absolutes can be stated at this time.

In general, however, data generally supports the notion that most people already take in more inflammatory causing fats and preformed AA than is healthy, and not enough omega–3 fats in the form of fish oils, flax, etc. So, adding additional AA in the form of a supplement may not conducive to overall health and well-being.

There are simply more questions here then answers. Would a gram (1000 mg) of AA per day given to a healthy athlete do them any real harm? What if they take additional omega–3 with it in an attempt to counter some of the negative effects? Is the reputation of foods such as red meat and whole eggs as muscle builders due to their AA content? The answer to all of those questions is unknown.

All things taken together, including the fact that the only study looking directly at the effects of AA on strength trained men found essentially no benefits, AA must get a thumbs down from me at this time.

References

M. Roberts, C. Kerksick, L. Taylor, et al. Performance and body composition changes after 50 days of concomitant Arachidonic acid supplementation and resistance training. JISSN. 3 (1)S1-S29.2006.

Simopoulos AP. Evolutionary aspects of diet, the omega–6/omega–3 ratio and genetic variation: nutritional implications for chronic diseases. Biomed Pharmacother. 2006 Nov;60(9):502-507.

Simopoulos AP. The importance of the ratio of omega–6/omega–3 essential fatty acids. Biomed Pharmacother. 2002 Oct;56(8):365-79.

Trappe TA, White F, Lambert CP, et al. Effect of ibuprofen and acetaminophen on postexercise muscle protein synthesis. Am J Physiol Endocrinol Metab. 2002 Mar;282(3):E551-6.

Trappe TA, Fluckey JD, White F, et al. Skeletal muscle PGF(2)(alpha) and PGE(2) in response to eccentric resistance exercise: influence of ibuprofen acetaminophen. J Clin Endocrinol Metab. 2001 Oct;86(10):5067-70.

ф

CREATINE MONOHYDRATE

What is it?

Creatine is formed in the human body from the amino acids methionine, glycine, and arginine. Creatine is stored in the human body as creatine phosphate (CP) or phosphocreatine. The average person's body contains approximately 120 grams of creatine stored as creatine and creatine phosphate.

Creatine can also be supplied by foods. Certain foods such as beef, herring, and salmon, are fairly high in creatine, but a person would have to eat pounds of these foods daily to equal what can be found in one teaspoon of powdered creatine from a supplement.

What is it supposed to do?

During short maximal bouts of exercise such as weight training or sprinting, stored adenosine triphosphate (ATP) is the dominant energy source. However, stored ATP is depleted rapidly. To give energy, ATP loses a phosphate and becomes adenosine diphosphate (ADP). At this point, the ADP must be converted back to ATP to derive energy from this energy producing system.

When ATP is depleted, it can be recharged by creatine, in the form of creatine phosphate. That is, the CP donates a phosphate to the ADP making it ATP again. An increased pool of CP means faster and greater recharging of ATP and, therefore, more work can be performed for a short duration, such as sprinting, weight lifting and other explosive anaerobic endeavors.

Other effects of creatine may be increases in protein synthesis and increased cell hydration, though researchers are still elucidating the mechanisms.

What does the research say for athletic performance?

The above is, of course, an immensely oversimplified review of an exceptionally complex system, but the basic explanation is correct. To date, research has shown ingesting creatine can increase the total body pool of CP which leads to greater generation of force with anaerobic forms of exercise, such as weight training, sprinting, etc.

Early research with creatine showed it can increase lean body mass and improve performance in sports that require high intensity intermittent exercise such as sprinting, weight lifting, football, etc.

Creatine has had spotty results in research that examined its effects on endurance oriented sports such as swimming, rowing and long distance running, with some studies showing no positive effects on performance with endurance athletes. Whether or not the failure of creatine to improve performance with endurance athletes was due to the nature of the sport or the design of the studies is still being debated. But one thing is for sure; the research is stronger in high intensity sports of short duration.

Recent findings with creatine monohydrate have confirmed previous research showing it's a safe and effective supplement. More recent research has focused on exactly how it works, and has looked deeper into its potential medical uses. Several studies have shown it can reduce cholesterol by up to 15%, and may be useful for treating wasting syndromes such as HIV. Creatine is also being looked at as a supplement that may help with diseases affecting the neuromuscular system, such as muscular dystrophy (MS) and others.

A plethora of recent studies suggest creatine may have therapeutic applications in aging populations, muscle atrophy, fatigue, gyrate atrophy, Parkinson's disease, Huntington's disease, and other mitochondrial cytopathies, neuropathic disorders, dystrophies, myopathies and brain pathologies.

The importance of creatine is underscored by creatine deficiency disorders: inborn errors of metabolism that prevent creatine from being manufactured. People born without the enzyme(s) responsible for making creatine suffer from a variety of neurological and developmental symptoms which are mitigated with creatine supplementation.

As for safety, some have suggested that creatine might increase the need for extra fluid intake to avoid potential dehydration and muscle pulls. Still, creatine has not been shown to increase either dehydration or muscle pulls in the research. In some people, creatine may increase a by-product of creatine metabolism called creatinine, which is a crude indicator but not a cause of kidney problems.

Some doctors have mistakenly thought that high creatinine levels (in athletes using creatine) are a sign of kidney problems, but that is not the case. Creatinine is not toxic to the kidneys and most doctors are not aware that creatine may raise creatinine levels with no toxicity to the kidneys. People with pre-existing kidney problems might want to avoid creatine due to the effects it can have on this test, though creatine supplementation has never been shown to be toxic to the kidneys and the vast number, of studies to date have found creatine to be exceedingly safe.

It's interesting to note that there has been a concerted effort by many groups and ignorant medical professionals to portray creatine as being somehow poorly researched (flatly untrue) and unsafe for long term use. They systematically ignore the dozens of studies that exist showing it's both safe and effective. Even more bizarre, they ignore the recent studies that are finding creatine may help literally thousands of people with the aforementioned diseases.

This is unscientific, unethical, and just plain immoral, in my view.

One question that often comes up regarding creatine is whether or not the loading phase is required. Originally, the advice for getting optimal results was to load up on creatine followed by a maintenance dose thereafter. This advice was based on the fact that the human body already contains approximately 120 grams of creatine (as creatine and creatine phosphate) stored in tissues and to increase total creatine stores, one had to load for several days in order to increase those stores above those levels.

The idea also seemed to work well, in practice, with people noticing considerable increases in strength and weight during the loading phase. All was not perfect however as many people found the loading phase to be a problem, with gastrointestinal upset, diarrhea and other problems. At the very least, loading was inconvenient and potentially expensive.

The need for a loading phase was a long held belief, but is it really needed to derive the benefits of creatine? The answer appears to be no, as both research and real world experience have found the loading phase may not be needed after all. A 1996 study compared a loading phase vs. no loading phase among 31 male subjects. The subjects loaded for 6 days using 20 g/day and a maintenance dose 2 g/day for a further 30 days. As expected, tissue creatine levels went up approximately 20 percent and the participants got stronger and gained lean mass. Nothing new there! And, not surprisingly, without a maintenance dose creatine levels went back to normal after 30 days.

Then the group was given 3g of creatine without a loading dose. The study found a similar—but more gradual—increase in muscle creatine concentrations over a period of 28 days. The researchers concluded:

" ...a rapid way to creatine load human skeletal muscle is to ingest 20 g of creatine for 6 days. This elevated tissue concentration can then be maintained by ingestion of 2 g/day thereafter. The ingestion of 3 g creatine/day is, in the long term, likely to be as effective at raising tissue levels as this higher dose."

A more recent study done in 1999 found that 5 g of creatine per day without a loading phase in 16 athletes significantly increased measures of strength, power, and increased body mass without a change in body fat levels (whereas the placebo group showed no significant changes).

The researcher of this 1999 study concluded:

" ...these data also indicate that lower doses of creatine monohydrate may be ingested (5 g/d), without a short–term, large–dose loading phase (20 g/d), for an extended period to achieve significant performance enhancement."

So, if you have suffered through the loading phase in the past thinking it was the only way to maximize the effects of your creatine supplement, it appears you can rest assured you don't have to go through all that hassle. A 3 to 5 gram per day dose over an extended period of time will probably do the same thing.

What about real world athletic performance?

What can I say? Creatine monohydrate is one of the most widely used supplements in bodybuilding, and I know of very few people who feel that they haven't gotten good results from using it.

Will Brink's Recommendation

Creatine can be found in the form of creatine monohydrate (CM), creatine citrate, creatine phosphate, tri–creatine malate, creatine–magnesium chelate and even liquid "creatine serum" to name just a few of the "high tech" versions competing with CM. The newest form being touted as the best invention since the discovery of testosterone is creatine ethyl ester. However, the vast majority of research to date showing creatine effects on muscle mass and performance used the monohydrate form and most creatine found in supplements is in the monohydrate form.

There are many and surprisingly complicated problems with the above forms, but I will do my best to cover the essential issues. For one thing, these forms have little or no research supporting any of their claims, some of which are either totally outlandish, or biologically impossible. Many companies selling these products make claims, for example, that creatine monohydrate is poorly absorbed and or poorly metabolized by the body. This is simply untrue: research has found that creatine monohydrate is highly absorbable. Some claim less "bloating" or other supposed effects of monohydrate, but don't have a drop of data to support the claim, or even a feasible theory as to why their form would not have the effect vs. the monohydrate form.

They often claim dramatically improved absorption over monohydrate (without data), fewer side effects (without data), the ability to reduce the number of non-responders to creatine (without data), etc. Are you starting to see a theme here?!

Now, it's not impossible for example, that a creatine citrate or malate (both of which are simply creatine bound to a TCA cycle intermediate) may work for a higher percentage of people than the monohydrate form, thus reducing the number of non responders, but it has yet to be proven.

It may be that the creatine–magnesium chelate form—the most interesting form of the group in my view—may be superior to the monohydrate form for adding LBM or strength, but there has yet to be a single head–to–head study that compared one version to the other. That people are getting some results from these new forms is all well and fine, but are those results above and beyond that of monohydrate?

If so, is it simply from the malate, citrate, or magnesium? If a study was to find that an equal amount of creatine–malate, citrate, etc. was 10% more effective than monohydrate, but was 4 times as expensive, would you get the same results just taking a little more monohydrate? The answer to all those questions, which must be answered to recommend using any of these new forms, is (drum roll) unknown.

So, here we have what may be the most well researched supplement known to mankind (the monohydrate form), that has been shown to be cheap, safe, and effective, and people clamor for more expensive, poorly researched forms (e.g., malate, citrate, etc.), because some supplement companies tell them it's superior to the monohydrate form! Now, if people want to spend their money on other forms of creatine, there is nothing wrong with that per se, but they should at no time be under the impression (no matter how much the supplement company selling it claims) that what they are buying has been proven to be superior to the monohydrate form.

For increases in strength, LBM, and performance, creatine monohydrate gets an enthusiastic thumbs up.

References

Brewer GJ and Wallimann TW. Protective effect of the energy precursor creatine against toxicity of glutamate and beta–amyloid in rat hippocampal neurons. J Neurochem. 2000 May;74(5):1968–78.

Earnest CP, Almada AL, and Mitchell TL. High–performance capillary electrophoresis–pure Creatine monohydrate reduces blood lipids in men and women. Clin Sci (Lond). 1996 Jul;91(1):113-8.

Ferrante RJ, Andreassen OA, Jenkins BG, et al. Neuroprotective effects of creatine in a transgenic mouse model of Huntington's disease. J Neurosci. 2000 Jun 15;20(12):4389-97.

Hultman E, Soderlund K, Timmons JA, et al. Muscle creatine loading in men.J Appl Physiol. 1996 Jul;81(1):232-7.

Klivenyi P, Ferrante RJ, Matthews RT, et al. Neuroprotective effects of creatine in a transgenic animal model of amyotrophic lateral sclerosis. Nat Med. 1999 Mar;5(3):347-50.

Kreider RB, Ferreira M, Wilson M, et al. Effects of creatine supplementation on body composition, strength, and sprint performance. Med Sci Sports Exerc. 1998 Jan;30(1):73-82.

Malcon C, Kaddurah–Daouk R, Beal MF. Neuroprotective effects of creatine administration against NMDA and malonate toxicity. Brain Res. 2000 Mar 31;860(1-2):195-8.

Matthews RT, Yang L, Jenkins BG, et al. Neuroprotective effects of creatine and cyclocreatine in animal models of Huntington's disease. J Neurosci. 1998 Jan 1;18(1):156–63.

Matthews RT, Ferrante RJ, Klivenyi P, et al. Creatine and cyclocreatine attenuate MPTP neurotoxicity. Exp Neurol. 1999 May;157(1):142-9.

Odland LM, MacDougall JD, Tarnopolsky MA, et al. Effect of oral creatine supplementation on muscle [PCr] and short–term maximum power output. Med Sci Sports Exerc. 1997 Feb;29(2):216-9.

Pearson DR, Hamby DG, et al. Long–term effects of Creatine monohydrate on strength and power. J Strength Cond Res. 1999 13(3):187-92.

Peeters BM, Lantz CD and Mayhew JL. Effect of oral creatine monohydrate and creatine phosphate supplementation on maximal strength indices, body composition, and blood pressure. J Strength Cond Res. 1999 13(1):3-9.

Poortmans JR, Auquier H, Renaut V, et al. Effect of short–term creatine supplementation on renal responses in men. Eur J Appl Physiol Occup Physiol. 1997;76(6):566-7.

Poortmans JR, Francaux M. Long–term oral creatine supplementation does not impair renal function in healthy athletes. Med Sci Sports Exerc. 1999 Aug;31(8):1108-10.

Tarnopolsky M, Martin J. Creatine monohydrate increases strength in patients with neuromuscular disease. Neurology. 1999 Mar 10;52(4):854-7

Volek JS, Duncan ND, Mazzetti SA, et al. No Effect of Heavy Resistance Training and Creatine Supplementation on Blood Lipids. Int J Sport Nutr Exerc Metab. 2000 Jun;10(2):144-56.

Walter MC, Lochmuller H, Reilich P, et al. Creatine monohydrate in muscular dystrophies: A double–blind, placebo–controlled clinical study. Neurology. 2000 May 9;54(9):1848-50.

☧

CARNITINE

What is it?

L–carnitine is often referred to as an "amino acid like" substance. The body synthesizes carnitine from the amino acids L–lysine and L–methionine. High levels of carnitine can be found in animal meats, especially red meats, from cows, lamb, and sheep.

Carnitine supplements come in a number of different forms. The most common are L–carnitine–L–tartrate, acetyl–L–carnitine, and propionyl–L–carnitine.

What is it supposed to do?

Carnitine has many functions in the human body, but is best known for its ability to shuttle long chain fatty acids across the membrane of cells so they can be burned (oxidized) for energy by the mitochondria.

Mitochondria are often referred to as the "power house" of cells where energy is produced. The actual process of how carnitine shuttles fatty acids to the mitochondria is fairly complex and detailed. Suffice it to say, it involves several enzymes and steps before the fats you want to burn end up being utilized by the mitochondria. So, the carnitine shuttle system is essential for the body to be able to burn fats as energy and this is why companies sell carnitine as a "fat burner."

What does the research say for athletic performance?

Studies that have focused on weight loss in people using carnitine as a supplement are few and conflicting. There are far more studies that look at carnitine as a sports and energy enhancing supplement, with some studies suggesting carnitine may help endurance athletes.

In animals, some studies have found increases in the use of fat for energy with high dose carnitine supplementation, but human studies are mixed, with some showing effects on endurance while others find no effect.

The difference may be dose and or the nutritional status of the athletes being tested. Doses used are generally high, in the 2 to 5 g range and higher.

Carnitine does appear to have real health uses and is even listed in the *Physicians Desk Reference* (a.k.a. the PDR) for certain pathologies involving the heart. Many alternative doctors swear by it for that use.

Carnitine may also help reduce cholesterol and increase HDL cholesterol, the "good" cholesterol. Acetyl–L–carnitine in particular has potential uses as an "anti–aging" supplement.

A number of animal experiments have shown improvements in mitochondrial function reduced by aging. It also appears to have neuroprotective and cognitive effects. Both acetyl–L–carnitine and propionyl–L–carnitine have been used as experimental therapies for erectile dysfunction and fatigue associated with male aging.

There are a couple of studies that indicate L–carnitine might have some uses for recovery. In one study, untrained subjects taking 3 g of L–carnitine/day for 3 weeks, experienced less muscle damage and pain following a session of eccentric exercise, relative to a placebo group. In the second study, recreationally weight trained men receiving 2 g of L–carnitine–L–tartrate/day for 3 weeks showed less muscle damage after performing a squat protocol (5 sets x 15-20 reps).

Recent resurgence in interest in carnitine for athletes is due to several studies that found Glycine Propionyl-L-Carnitine (GPLC) improved performance, but effects have been somewhat contradictory in nature. For example, one study found at a dose of 4.5 g, GPLC actually had adverse effects on peak power (PP) and mean power (MP) compared to baseline values! At a lower dose tested however. (1.5 g /day), GPLC showed modest improvements in PP and MP (PP increased 3-6% while MP improved 2-5%) were observed compared to baseline values.

What about real world athletic performance?

L–carnitine has been disappointing as a fat loss nutrient. Acetyl–L–carnitine has a reputation as a "nootropic", and some swear by it for improving overall mood and focus. I do not know anyone who has tried carnitine as a recovery nutrient, so feedback on this use is lacking.

Will Brink's Recommendation

Although it may very well have potential health benefits in certain people, carnitine's performance improving and "fat burning" abilities are questionable.

People who wish to try carnitine will need to use at least 500 mg for more several times daily, with some studies using 5 g to 6 g (5000 mg–6000 mg) or more, daily.

While it is often found as an ingredient in weight loss formulas, people would be wise however to check the dose in such formulas as higher doses are clearly needed for any effect.

For general health and other uses, carnitine gets a thumbs up, but for building muscle it gets a thumbs down. For possibly improving endurance, it may be worth a try, albeit an expensive try if you follow the doses used in the studies.

References

Jacobs PL, et al. Long-term glycine propionyl-l-carnitine supplemention and paradoxical effects on repeated anaerobic sprint performance. J Int Soc Sports Nutr. 2010 Oct 28;7:35.

Jacobs PL et al. Glycine propionyl-L-carnitine produces enhanced anaerobic work capacity with reduced lactate accumulation in resistance trained males. J Int Soc Sports Nutr. 2009 Apr 2;6:9.

Vermeulen RC, Scholte HR. Exploratory open label, randomized study of acetyl- and propionylcarnitine in chronic fatigue syndrome. Psychosom Med. 2004 Mar-Apr;66(2):276-82.

Hiatt WR, Regensteiner JG, Creager MA, Hirsch AT, Cooke JP, Olin JW, Gorbunov GN, Isner J, Lukjanov YV, Tsitsiashvili MS, Zabelskaya TF, Amato A. Propionyl-L-carnitine improves exercise performance and functional status in patients with claudication. Am J Med. 2001 Jun 1;110(8):616-22.

Askew EW, Dohm GL, Weiser PC, et al. Supplemental dietary carnitine and lipid metabolism in exercising rats. Nutr Metab. 1980;24(1):32–42.

Giamberardino MA, Dragani L, Valente R, et al. Effects of prolonged L–carnitine administration on delayed muscle pain and CK release after eccentric effort. Int J Sports Med. 1996 Jul;17(5):320-4.

Gorostiaga EM, Maurer CA, Eclache JP. Decrease in respiratory quotient during exercise following L–carnitine supplementation. Int J Sports Med. 1989 Jun;10(3):169-74.

Kraemer WJ, Volek JS, French DN, et al. The effects of L–carnitine L–tartrate supplementation on hormonal responses to resistance exercise and recovery. J Strength Cond Res. 2003 Aug;17(3):455-62.

Soop M, Bjorkman O, Cederblad G, et al. Influence of carnitine supplementation on muscle substrate and carnitine metabolism during exercise. J Appl Physiol. 1988 Jun;64(6):2394-9.

Vecchiet L, Di Lisa F, Pieralisi G et al. Influence of L–carnitine administration on maximal physical exercise. Eur J Appl Physiol Occup Physiol. 1990;61(5-6):486-90.

℞

DHEA

What is it?

Dehydroepiandrosterone (DHEA) is a hormone produced primarily in the adrenal glands with minor amounts produced by the testes. It is found in both men and women. DHEA is the most abundant steroid hormone in the human body, and like all steroid hormones, ultimately comes from cholesterol. Most DHEA in the body is found as DHEA–sulfate (DHEA–S). DHEA is a major precursor to other steroid hormones, which is why some companies market it as a "muscle builder."

What is it supposed to do?

DHEA is marketed as being helpful for just about every human ailment from memory loss to heart disease to immune enhancement to weight loss, and more.

What does the research have to say?

DHEA consistently makes rodents such as mice and rats lose weight. In red eyed rodents (i.e. mice and rats), DHEA causes many biochemical changes that just don't seem to happen in people, showing just how different rats and people can be.

In people, the research has been far less impressive. Several studies using over 1500 mg per day of DHEA showed either no effects or short-lived effects on body composition in humans.

One early study found 1600 mg per day of DHEA (which is a very high dose of DHEA) reduced body fat and increased muscle mass in men, with later studies done by the same group and others failing to find that effect. Another study conducted in 1999 confirmed that supplementation of 150 mg/day DHEA for 8 weeks, in combination with a resistance training program had no effect on testosterone levels, strength, or lean mass in younger men. This result was echoed by a different research group, that found 100 mg/day DHEA resulted in small, non–significant increases in strength and lean mass in middle-aged, strength training men over a 12 week period.

Some studies in people using DHEA have shown slight increases in testosterone and insulin–like growth factor 1 (IGF–1) levels, but most studies—such as the one cited above—have found minimal effect in younger people. On the other hand, older people—particularly post–menopausal women—tend to show more improvement with DHEA supplementation. One recent study found that DHEA therapy enhanced the improvements seen with strength training with older adults.

The researchers concluded:

" DHEA alone for 6 mo did not significantly increase strength or thigh muscle volume. However, DHEA therapy potentiated the effect of 4 mo. of weightlifting training on muscle strength...and on thigh muscle volume...Serum insulin–like growth factor concentration increased in response to DHEA replacement. This study provides evidence that DHEA replacement has the beneficial effect of enhancing the increases in muscle mass and strength induced by heavy resistance exercise in elderly individuals. "

The research showing health improvements, such as cognitive benefits, immune enhancement, stress reduction, and anti-cancer benefits, is also compelling.

What about real world athletic performance?

I have known many people who genuinely felt DHEA helped them in many ways, including an improved feeling of well-being, but none of them claimed to have lost any weight using it. In my personal experiences with people over the years, no one has gained muscle, increased strength, or lost measurable amounts of body fat from the use of DHEA.

Will Brink's Recommendation

It's well known that DHEA levels fall off as we age, and the research on health uses of DHEA justifies using small amounts to counter this age related drop off, or deficiencies from other causes.

As a muscle building supplement in young healthy athletes, DHEA is almost certainly worthless, and high intakes may in fact be counterproductive to gaining muscle. Positive effects of DHEA in older individuals is much clearer, however, with only 25-100 mg per day needed to positively effect bone mineral density, lean mass, and body fat levels in older men and women.

Why the difference between old and young people?

DHEA and DHEA–S levels are one of the best biological markers of aging known. DHEA levels rise slowly till they peak at around 30 years of age, and decline steadily after age 35, with levels reduced by 70-80% by age 75. This effect is one of the most consistent and predictable changes in aging people known so far.

Though the utility of DHEA in younger people with normal physiological levels of DHEA is debatable, the benefits clearly outweigh any small risks in people over 40 who have reduced DHEA levels. Only blood tests will tell a person what their DHEA/DHEA–S levels are and where they are compared to others in their age group.

People interested in using DHEA as a general health benefiting supplement, should have blood tests done to determine their levels of DHEA/DHEA–S before using this supplement. For general DHEA replacement, very small amounts are needed, like 25-50 mg a day for men and even less for women.

As a bodybuilding supplement, it's generally been a bust. Also, though fairly safe, it's not an innocuous substance. DHEA is a steroid hormone and weak androgen. Some women have noticed increases in facial hair growth from using large amounts of DHEA.

References

Brown GA, Vukovich MD, Sharp RL, et al. Effect of oral DHEA on serum testosterone and adaptations to resistance training in young men. J Appl Physiol. 1999 Dec;87(6):2274-83.

Nestler JE, Barlascini CO, Clore JN, Blackard WG. Dehydroepiandrosterone reduces serum low density lipoprotein levels and body fat but does not alter insulin sensitivity in normal men. J Clin Endocrinol Metab. 1988 Jan;66(1):57-61.

Nissen SL, Sharp RL. Effect of dietary supplements on lean mass and strength gains with resistance exercise: a meta–analysis. J Appl Physiol. 2003 Feb;94(2):651-9.

Villareal DT, Holloszy JO. DHEA enhances effects of weight training on muscle mass and strength in elderly women and men. Am J Physiol Endocrinol Metab. 2006 Nov;291(5):E1003-8.

Wallace MB, Lim J, Cutler A, Bucci L. Effects of dehydroepiandrosterone vs. androstenedione supplementation in men. Med Sci Sports Exerc. 1999 Dec;31(12):1788-92.

♄

7–KETO DHEA

What is it?

7–Keto DHEA is 3–Acetyl–7–oxo–dehydroepiandrosterone—a naturally occurring metabolite of the steroid precursor DHEA.

What is it supposed to do?

7–Keto DHEA can allegedly provide many of the benefits of DHEA, without the drawbacks. It's marketed primarily as a fat loss supplement.

What does the research say for athletic performance?

As most people know, DHEA is claimed to help just about every ailment known to man kind, from depression, to heart disease, to cancer, to weight loss. The criticism of DHEA has been its potential effects on people's hormones, as DHEA can be converted into the sex hormones such as testosterone, estrogen, as well as others. Though research has been contradictory regarding DHEA's effects on hormones, most agree that it does have the potential for problems, if used in high enough doses.

Researchers looked into the possibility that there may be a downstream metabolite of DHEA that was responsible for many of its potentially positive effects on health without the downsides mentioned above. That metabolite appears to be 3–Acetyl–7–oxo–dehydroepiandrosterone, or simply 7–Keto DHEA. 7–Keto DHEA may in fact be more biologically active, that is have enhanced effects above that of DHEA, without the ability to alter hormone levels in the body of people using it.

In vitro (test tube) studies with 7–Keto DHEA appear to show it has no effects on steroid hormones and does not convert to sex hormones such as testosterone, estrogens, etc. One study that fed

200 mg of 7–Keto DHEA to men aged 18 – 49 years old for four weeks found no effects on sex hormone levels.

Interestingly, 7–Keto DHEA may have a more pronounced thermogenic effect (the 7–Keto DHEA process the body uses to convert stored calories into energy) than DHEA and a few animal studies and in vitro studies have shown this. However, no studies to date, in people, have looked specifically at the thermogenic effect of 7–Keto DHEA vs. DHEA. Some animal research has also shown improvements in memory and other cognitive functions. 7–Keto DHEA may also have positive effects on thyroid function.

One of the better known claims of DHEA is as a weight loss agent, but studies using various doses of DHEA for weight loss have been disappointing for the most part.

As for 7–Keto DHEA, there has been one recent study with people that looked at weight loss. The study fed 30 overweight women (15 acted as a control group and received a placebo) 200 mg a day of 7–Keto DHEA for 8 weeks. The study participants were put on a three–day per week cross training exercise program. The study found that the group getting the 7–Keto DHEA lost 1.8 percent of its body weight—a little over 6 lb on average —vs. the placebo group, that only lost 0.57 percent of its body weight. The study also found that the group getting the 7–Keto DHEA had increases in the thyroid hormone T3, without significant changes in testosterone, estradiol (estrogen), liver and kidney function tests, blood sugar vital signs, or overall caloric intake over the eight week study.

There were no adverse effects reported throughout the study in the people getting the 7–Keto–DHEA supplement.

The study concluded:

" 200 mg of 7–Keto–DHEA per day yields a significant reduction in both body weight and body fat. "

However, it's important to note that this is just one small human study and more research is clearly needed.

On paper, 7–Keto DHEA looks promising. We do have some human research regarding weight loss, albeit only one study. The study is a compelling one however, and appears to show 7–Keto DHEA has effects that are different from that of simple DHEA on weight loss, though more human studies are clearly needed.

What about real world athletic performance?

Feedback on 7–Keto DHEA alone as a fat loss agent has been lackluster. It gets more favorable notice as part of a stack.

Will Brink's Recommendation

7–Keto DHEA should be a very safe supplement, though it probably will not be a supplement that improves athletic prowess. As people know, both DHEA and 7–Keto are often touted for building muscle or improving performance, but there is no data to show that with 7–Keto, and data with DHEA are conflicting at best.

For general health and possibly weight loss, 7–Keto gets a tentative thumbs up, but for increasing muscle mass, strength, or performance, it gets a thumbs down (as does DHEA) at this time.

References

Colker MD, Torina G, Swain MA, Kalman DS. Double–Blind, Placebo–Controlled, Randomized Clinical Trial Evaluating the Effects of Exercise Plus 3–Acetyl–7–oxo–dehydroepiandrosterone on Body Composition and the Endocrine System in Overweight Adults. JEPonline 1999 2(4).

Lardy H, Kneer N, Bellei M, Bobyleva V. Induction of thermogenic enzymes by DHEA and its metabolites. Ann N Y Acad Sci. 1995 Dec 29;774:171-9.

Lardy H, Kneer N, Wei Y, et al. Ergosteroids. II: Biologically active metabolites and synthetic derivatives of dehydroepiandrosterone. Steroids. 1998 Mar;63(3):158-65. Erratum in: Steroids 1999 Jul;64(7):497.

ф

GABA

What is it?

Gamma–aminobutyric acid (GABA) is primary inhibitory neurotransmitter found in the brain and is produced from glutamate and vitamin B6, via the enzymes L–glutamic acid decarboxylase and pyridoxal phosphate. There are neurotransmitters that cause excitation in the brain and there are neurotransmitters that have the opposite effect. The balance between excitatory and inhibitory neurotransmitters is essential to proper brain function and has direct effects on all facets of human physiology, mood, health, and well-being.

This is an intensive and ongoing area of research far beyond the scope of this book.

What is it supposed to do?

Because GABA is an inhibitory neurotransmitter, it's associated with inducing relaxation, reducing stress, and as a sleep aid. For example, drugs in benzodiazepine family (e.g., Xanax, etc.) have been shown to induce relaxation by stimulating GABA receptors, and hence induce relaxation. There's a long list of drugs hat work by interacting with GABA receptors (GABA receptor agonists) or act by increasing levels of GABA in the brain, with varying effects.

This is an extremely simplified explanation for an incredibly complex—and not fully understood—system, but it will have to suffice for this section. As a supplement, GABA has a reputation for improving sleep and causing mild relaxation. Particular to the interests of bodybuilders and other athletes, GABA has been sold as a growth hormone (GH) releaser due to GABA's known role as a modulator of GH release.

What does the research say for athletic performance?

As the claims regarding the effects of GABA as a supplement are varied, I will stick to its supposed effects on GH. Some human and animal studies suggest GABA can increase GH levels. For example, a recent study carried out at the University of Shizuoka in Japan, found GABA increased GH output in rats as well as having statistically significant effects on other measures, such a increased protein synthetic rates in the rats brain, liver and gastrocnemius muscle. Doses used were quite high: the most effective oral dose was between 50 mg and 100 mg/100 g body weight GABA.

To which they concluded:

" Our results suggest that the treatment of GABA to young male rats are likely to increase the concentrations of plasma GH and the rate of protein synthesis in the brain, and that RNA activity is at least partly related to the fractional rate of brain protein synthesis."

On the human side of things, an older study found GABA had statistically significant effects on the GH levels of 19 men given 5 g of GABA orally with 18 additional men given placebos. The study found that given as a single acute dose, GABA increased GH levels. However, a smaller group of 8 men given 18 g per day for four days were found to have a greatly blunted response to GH release and increased levels of the hormone prolactin. Leading them to conclude:

" These results indicate that pharmacological doses of GABA affect growth hormone and prolactin secretion in man. The precise nature of GABA's effects as well as its mechanism of action remains to be clarified."

There are essentially no modern studies that have replicated those finding in humans in vivo, although the animal study mentioned above was more recent.

What about real world athletic performance?

GABA is a supplement that has been around a long time. In all those years I have yet to meet anyone who noticed any significant effects on muscle mass, body fat, or performance using GABA. Some have reported mild sedative effects and improved sleep using GABA, but feedback has been mixed at best and data on those uses is also lacking.

Will Brink's Recommendation

Although GABA has been purported to increase levels of GH, studies that found the effect are either quite old and/or the results failed to be replicated in most cases. More importantly, it's unclear if GABA can even pass the blood–brain barrier, which selectively allows some things access to the brain while blocking others. What that means is GABA supplements are probably not an effective way to increase this neurotransmitter because it can't easily cross the blood–brain barrier.

Oddly, GABA is listed as being effective for treating all manner of human ailments, such as insomnia, stress, chronic pain, epilepsy, Fibromyalgia and tobacco withdrawal symptoms! There is no solid data to support the use of GABA for any of the above, though GABA appears to be quite safe. Typical doses range from as low as few hundred milligrams per day to multiple grams (2–5 g) taken several times per day.

I consider the issue of whether or not GABA actually increases GH to be a moot point. Bottom line, GABA may or may not affect GH; but affecting GH does not equal any effects on body composition anyway, as mentioned above; therefore GABA gets a "not worth using" recommendation from me at this time.

References

Acs Z, Lonart G, Makara GB. Role of hypothalamic factors (growth–hormone–releasing hormone and gamma–aminobutyric acid) in the regulation of growth hormone secretion in the neonatal and adult rat. Neuroendocrinology. 1990 Aug;52(2):156-60.

Cavagnini F, Benetti G, Invitti C, Ramella G, et al. Effect of gamma–aminobutyric acid on growth hormone and prolactin secretion in man: influence of pimozide and domperidone. J Clin Endocrinol Metab. 1980 Oct;51(4):789-92.

Cavagnini F, Invitti C, Pinto M, Maraschini C, et al. Effect of acute and repeated administration of gamma aminobutyric acid (GABA) on growth hormone and prolactin secretion in man. Acta Endocrinol (Copenh). 1980 Feb;93(2):149-54.

Koulu M, Lammintausta R, Dahlstrom S. Effects of some gamma–aminobutyric acid (GABA)–ergic drugs on the dopaminergic control of human growth hormone secretion. J Clin Endocrinol Metab. 1980 Jul;51(1):124-9.

McCann SM, Vijayan E, Negro–Vilar A, et al. Gamma aminobutyric acid (GABA), a modulator of anterior pituitary hormone secretion by hypothalamic and pituitary action. Psychoneuroendocrinology. 1984;9(2):97–106.

Mezo I, Kovacs M, Szoke B, Szabo EZ, et al. New Gaba–containing analogues of human growth hormone–releasing hormone (1-30)–amide: I. Synthesis and in vitro biological activity. J Endocrinol Invest. 1993 Nov;16(10):793-8.

Monteleone P, Maj M, Iovino M, Steardo L. Evidence for a sex difference in the basal growth hormone response to GABAergic stimulation in humans. Acta Endocrinol (Copenh). 1988 Nov;119(3):353-7.

Murakami Y, Kato Y, Kabayama Y, Tojo K, et al. Involvement of growth hormone–releasing factor in growth hormone secretion induced by gamma–aminobutyric acid in conscious rats. Endocrinology. 1985 Aug;117(2):787-9.

Spencer GS, Berry CJ, Bass JJ. Neuroendocrine regulation of growth hormone secretion in sheep. VII. Effects of GABA. Regul Pept. 1994 Aug 4;52(3):181-6.

Steardo L, Iovino M, Monteleone P, et al. Evidence for a GABAergic control of the exercise–induced rise in GH in man. Eur J Clin Pharmacol. 1985; 28(5):607-9.

Steardo L, Iovino M, Monteleone P, et al. Pharmacological evidence for a dual GABAergic regulation of growth hormone release in humans. Life Sci. 1986 Sep 15;39(11):979-85.

Tujioka K, Okuyama S, Yokogoshi H, Fukaya Y, et al. Dietary gamma–aminobutyric acid affects the brain protein synthesis rate in young rats. Amino Acids. 2007 Feb;32(2):255-60.

Zarandi M, Serfozo P, Zsigo J, Deutch AH, et al. Potent agonists of growth hormone–releasing hormone. II. Pept Res. 1992 Jul–Aug;5(4):190-3.

☧

HMB AND KIC

What are they?

"HMB" is beta–hydroxymethylbutyric acid; "KIC" is alpha–ketoisocaproic acid. Both are metabolites of the amino acid leucine, which plays a key role in protein synthesis. L–leucine is one of three amino acids known as the branched chain amino acids or BCAA (isoleucine and valine being the other two). KIC and HMB are intermediates in the oxidative breakdown of leucine, where it is deaminated and converted first into KIC, then into HMB. Eventually, the carbon skeleton is converted to acetyl–CoA, and enters the citric acid (Krebs) cycle to be used for energy production.

What are they supposed to do?

As sports supplements, they're marketed as anti-catabolics. Rather than increasing LBM by enhancing protein synthesis, they work by decreasing protein breakdown. HMB has been promoted more aggressively, and is better known than KIC.

What does the research say for athletic performance?

HMB appears to be one of those classic supplements that looks great in the lab but has had a rocky track record with real world users. But let me back up a moment.

It has been known for a long time that BCAAs play a critical role in the turn over of lean body tissues (muscle) and is muscle sparing (i.e. anti-catabolic) in a variety of muscle wasting states. Of the three BCAAs, L–leucine appears to be the most important to preserving hard earned muscle mass, and intense exercise and certain disease states have been shown to eat up a great deal of L–leucine. So far so good!

The main drawback of L–leucine is the fact that you must use large amounts of this amino acid to get a positive effect, making it both expensive and impractical.

Many studies that showed benefits were in fact done intravenously and used as much as 5 grams per hour of L–leucine! That, my friend, is a lot of leucine. So, it was theorized there might be a metabolite of this ultra important amino acid that was responsible for many of the positive effects of L–leucine but could be taken in far lower doses and by mouth (as opposed to having a tube stuck in your arm). That metabolite appears to be HMB.

Animal research with HMB has been impressive. During stressful conditions, animals will often lose weight and/or become quite ill. Some even die. This of course can be quite expensive for any company trying to make a living from these animals in one way or another. When animals were fed HMB a large reduction in mortality rates, increases in muscle mass, and improvements in immune function were found.

Several studies in humans have also looked promising. Studies using both trained and untrained subjects found increases in muscle and decreases in body fat in people ingesting just three grams (3000 mg) of HMB per day.

The average was approximately 2–4 pounds of muscle put on with an equal amount of fat taken off over a four week period. The scientists also found that HMB positively affected several biochemical markers of intense exercise that would lead one to believe that there was a reduction of muscle wasting in people taking HMB.

"So what's the problem," you ask? The problem has been mainly that what looked so promising in the research has not been fully realized in the real world, hence my introduction to this section. Several follow up studies with HMB in people also failed to find any results.

Human research with KIC has been scanty. A recent study on glycine–arginine–alpha–ketoisocaproic acid (GAKIC) supplementation found it attenuated the decrease in mean power output between sprints in a bicycle ergometer test.

Another recent study found that a 14 day preload of HMB (3 g/day) and KIC (0.3 g/day) reduced some of the symptoms of muscle damage in untrained males after a single exercise session.

What about real world athletic performance?

Feedback from real world users has been generally negative with HMB. Some seem to feel they have benefited from it, while most found HMB a big waste of money. Even fewer feel they've derived any benefit from GAKIC, the current form of KIC on the market.

Were the studies that found benefits flawed? Are some people not taking enough? Does it depend on the nutritional status of the person using it and/or how they train?

It's not known for sure at this time, but considering the costs of HMB and GAKIC and the fact there are other less expensive alternatives that clearly work (i.e., creatine) I see no reason for hard working athletes to spend money on these supplements until a definitive answer can be found. At this time, both get a thumbs down for building muscle, but if you want to give them a try, I will not hold it against you.

References

Buckspan R, Hoxworth B, Cersosimo E, et al. Alpha–Ketoisocaproate is superior o leucine in sparing glucose utilization in humans. Am J Physiol. 1986 Dec;251(6 Pt 1):E648-53.

Buford BN, Koch AJ. Glycine–arginine–alpha–ketoisocaproic acid improves performance of repeated cycling sprints. Med Sci Sports Exerc. 2004 Apr; 36(4):583-7.

Mortimore GE, Poso AR, Kadowaki M, Wert JJ Jr. Multiphasic control of hepatic protein degradation by regulatory amino acids. General features and hormonal modulation. J Biol Chem. 1987 Dec 5;262(34):16322–7.

Flakoll PJ, VandeHaar MJ, Kuhlman G, Nissen S. Influence of alpha–ketoisocaproate on lamb growth, feed conversion, and carcass composition. J AnimSci. 1991 Apr;69(4):1461-7.

May ME, Buse MG. Effects of branched–chain amino acids on protein turnover. Diabetes Metab Rev. 1989 May;5(3):227-45.

Nair KS, Schwartz RG, Welle S. Leucine as a regulator of whole body and skeletal muscle protein metabolism in humans. Am J Physiol. 1992 Nov;263(5 Pt 1):E928-34.

Nissen S, Morrical D, Fuller JC. The effects of the leucine catabolite ß–hydroxy–ß–methylbutyrate on the growth and health of growing lambs. 1994 J Anim Sci. 77 (Suppl. 1):243.

Nissen S, Panton J, et al. Effects of ß–hydroxy ß–methylbutyrate (HMB) supplementation on strength and body composition of trained and untrained males undergoing intense resistance training. Experimental Biology Conference Presentation Abstract (1996).

Talleyrand V, Dorn A, et al. Effects of feeding ß–hydroxy ß–methylbutyrate on immune function in stressed calves. FASEB Journal 1994 (8), p. A951.

Van Koevering M, Nissen S. Oxidation of leucine and alpha–ketoisocaproate to beta–hydroxy–beta–methylbutyrate in vivo. Am J Physiol. 1992 Jan;262(1 Pt 1):E27-31.

Van Koevering MT, Dolezal HG, et al. Effects of beta–hydroxy–beta–methyl butyrate on performance and carcass quality of feedlot steers. J Anim Sci 1994 72: 1927-1935.

van Someren KA, Edwards AJ, Howatson G. Supplementation with beta–hydroxy–beta–methylbutyrate (HMB) and alpha–ketoisocaproic acid (KIC) reduces signs and symptoms of exercise-induced muscle damage in man. Int J Sport Nutr Exerc Metab. 2005 Aug;15(4):413-24.

ԃ

PHOSPHATIDYLSERINE

What is it?

Phosphatidylserine is a phospholipid found in cell membranes. It's composed of two fatty acids and the amino acid L–serine, linked to a glycerophosphate backbone; chemically, it's known as 1,2–diacyl–sn–glycerol–(3)–L–phosphoserine. It was first isolated from brain lipids called cephalins.

What is it supposed to do?

Supplemental phosphatidylserine may enhance cognitive function and suppress cortisol production.

What does the research say for athletic performance?

Phosphatidylserine (PS) is a supplement that has been found to hold great promise for people suffering from various pathologies that affect the brain, such as certain forms of dementia, Alzheimer's, and others. Early European studies showed phosphatidylserine could slow and reverse the rate of brain cell aging in laboratory animals.

PS also restored mental function in older animals to levels exceeding those found in some younger animals (although studies in humans with Alzheimer's disease were less impressive, PS still produced improvements in cognitive function). Research has shown that in addition to improving neural function, PS appears to enhance energy metabolism in brain cells. In the brain, PS helps maintain cell membrane integrity and may protect brain cells against the functional deterioration that occurs with "normal" aging.

Brain tissue has been found to be especially rich in PS and it appears aging causes a decline in the PS content of cells throughout the body. So, it's no wonder that longevity groups and individuals concerned with brain function due to various causes have taken an interest in PS.

One effect of PS may be its ability to reduce levels of the catabolic (muscle wasting) hormone cortisol after exercise. Two early studies done in Italy appeared to show that chronic intakes of PS reduced the release of cortisol after intense exercise. When the body senses stress, whether physical and/or emotional, it releases cortisol as part of the "fight or flight" cascade that prepares us for short term survival. Prolonged stress from malnutrition, surgery, overtraining and sleep deprivation, as well as psychological stress, causes a systemic effect that includes increased cortisol secretion resulting in a decline in certain aspects of the immune system and other problems.

As the reader can see, over long periods of time, high cortisol levels are detrimental to our overall health and muscle mass. A supplement that could reduce cortisol has obvious applications for athletes.

There is one catch: PS in supplements is usually derived from soy. Most of the aforementioned studies used PS derived from bovine cortex, which is not recommended for human consumption due to fear of contamination by the prions associated with Bovine Spongiform Encephalitis (BSE), or "Mad Cow Disease." The soy-derived PS is somewhat different than the bovine-derived version. PS from soy has mostly polyunsaturated fatty acids, whereas the fatty acids in bovine PS are a mixture of saturated and monounsaturated fatty acids, along with the essential fatty acid metabolite docosahexaenoic acid. There is some question, therefore, if soy-derived PS is as effective as the bovine version.

Several recent studies have shed some light on the subject. In one of them, 750 mg/day soy PS was found to significantly increase the time to exhaustion in a cycling trial, although two additional studies by the same group found that it did not reduce oxidative stress, markers of inflammation, muscle damage, perceived soreness, or cortisol levels following downhill or intermittent (sprint) running.

Another study, found 400 mg/day of soy PS was effective in blunting serum and salivary cortisol and emotional distress in response to psychological stress. It's not completely clear from the above studies if soy PS is equivalent to bovine PS, although there do appear to be some potential benefits to its use.

What about real world athletic performance?

Anecdotally, people who have tried PS report mild improvements to their mood. A few have mentioned that they feel able to work out longer as well. The doses most take range from 600–800 mg/day; few notice any results at lower doses.

Will Brink's Recommendation

PS does suffer from one key drawback; its sheer cost. The doses used in the latest studies range from 400–800 mg/day, while most supplements supply no more than 100 mg/capsule. Another drawback is that PS has not been studied to see whether or not it would truly improve either strength or muscle mass in athletes, which is ultimately the bottom line for recommending a product.

At this time, PS gets a very tentative thumbs up for athletes, but again, it's far from clear what effects it will have on muscle mass or performance, or what the optimal dose is.

References

Hellhammer J, Fries E, Buss C, et al. Effects of soy lecithin phosphatidic acid and phosphatidylserine complex (PAS) on the endocrine and psychological responses to mental stress. Stress. 2004 Jun;7(2):119-26.

Kelly GS. Nutritional and botanical interventions to assist with the adaptation to stress. Altern Med Rev. 1999 Aug;4(4):249–65.

Kingsley MI, Kilduff LP, McEneny J, et al. Phosphatidylserine supplementation and recovery following downhill running. Med Sci Sports Exerc. 2006 Sep;38(9):1617-25.

Kingsley MI, Miller M, Kilduff LP, et al. Effects of phosphatidylserine on exercise capacity during cycling in active males. Med Sci Sports Exerc. 2006 Jan;38(1):64-71.

Kingsley MI, Wadsworth D, Kilduff LP, et al. Effects of phosphatidylserine on oxidative stress following intermittent running. Med Sci Sports Exerc. 2005 Aug;37(8):1300-6.

Monteleone P, Maj M, Beinat L, et al. Blunting by chronic phosphatidylserine administration of the stress–induced activation of the hypothalamo–pituitary–adrenal axis in healthy men. Eur J Clin Pharmacol. 1992;42(4):385–8.

Monteleone P, Beinat L, Tanzillo C, et al. Effects of phosphatidylserine on the neuroendocrine response to physical stress in humans. Neuroendocrinology. 1990 Sep;52(3):243-8.

φ

RIBOSE

What is it?

Ribose is technically a sugar. There are many sugars the body uses for a wide variety of functions. Most people know about sugars such as glucose, sucrose, and fructose (blood sugar, table sugar and fruit sugar, respectively). For example, glucose can be found in some fruits and is the form of sugar found in the blood stream, hence the term "blood sugar."

Sucrose is often called "table sugar" as it is the common form added to many foods and is found in the sugar bowl on your table (sucrose is actually made up of glucose and fructose).

Fructose is often referred to as "fruit sugar" because it is found as the dominant sugar in fruit. There are however many other sugars the body uses for countless functions and/or is found in the foods we eat: xylose, galactose, lactose, mannose, ribose, and many others.

Ribose is widespread among all organisms and is a constituent of ribonucleic acid (RNA) which carries our genetic code. However, ribose is involved in many other functions in the body, including the production of high energy compounds the body uses to do work (i.e. exercise, etc.).

What is it supposed to do?

Data suggest that ribose may both serve as an energy source and enhance the production of compounds known as purine nucleotides. It is well established that high energy compounds such as ATP are reduced during and after intense exercise.

What does the research say for athletic performance?

The body must resynthesize these high energy compounds during the post-exercise recuperation phase and this is where ribose may come into play. By adding an external dietary source of ribose in high enough doses, athletes may be able to recuperate faster from intense workouts and thus can improve performance and strength. In studies where the normal synthesis of these high energy compounds is reduced by certain diseases or genetic problems, ribose has looked promising for helping people afflicted with such problems.

However, studies looking at healthy athletes showing improvements in strength or performance give mixed results. For example, a small study with 15 male bodybuilders examined exercise performance over a four week period.

The men were given 5 g of ribose before they performed the bench press and 5 g following the exercise vs. a group taking a placebo. The study found a statistically significant increase in the number of repetitions performed in the bench press in athletes getting the ribose compared to athletes taking the placebo (5 subjects in the ribose group and 7 in the placebo group).

The number of bench press repetitions performed to muscular failure increased +29.8% ribose vs. +7.42% placebo (p = 0.046) over the 4 week period. Another relatively small study with 16 athletes receiving 10 g of ribose and put through repeated sprints had an increase in mean power over 5 days of training (4.2% vs. 0.6%).

Findings also included greater peak power output at the last sprint session (11.4 watts/kg vs. 10.4 watts/kg, p=0.05 time) vs. a placebo group. However, it's important to note that these are both small studies and neither have been published in a peer reviewed journal (see references).

On the other hand, a study on 19 trained males taking 10 g ribose/day for 5 days showed modest improvements in total work output, but no improvements in anaerobic exercise capacity or differences in lactate, ammonia, and other metabolic markers.

Another study using 32 g ribose/day concluded:

" ...ribose supplementation did not show reproducible increases in performance across all 6 sprints. Therefore, within the framework of this investigation, it appears that ribose supplementation does not have a consistent or substantial effect on anaerobic cycle sprinting."

In yet another study, researchers measuring the effect of 16 g ribose /day on maximal exercise and ATP recovery following a series of dynamic knee extensions stated:

" Oral ribose supplementation with 4 g doses four times a day does not beneficially impact on postexercise muscle ATP recovery and maximal intermittent exercise performance."

Even a longer term study on rowing performance turned up negative. Members of a collegiate rowing team took 10 g ribose for 8 weeks before and after practice, while a control group took the same amount of dextrose. At the end of 8 weeks, the dextrose group showed greater improvements in timed trials than the ribose group.

What about real world athletic performance?

Ribose gets mixed reviews from people who've tried it. A few stack it with creatine and feel that there's some improvement. Others feel nothing at all.

Will Brink's Recommendation

Ribose is one of those supplements that look good in theory, but won't really do much in the real world application. It does appear to help people with various pathologies, but there's a lack of large scale human studies that are published in peer reviewed journals showing it will increase LBM, strength or performance. It's also fairly expensive. Overall, I have to give ribose a thumbs down at this point as there are better ways to spend your hard earned money.

References

Antonio J, Van Gammeren D, Falk D. The effects of ribose supplementation of exercise performance in recreational male bodybuilders. Data on file at Bioenergy, Inc., 13840 Johnson Street N.E., Ham Lake, Minnesota 55304 USA.

Berardi JM, Ziegenfuss TN. Effects of ribose supplementation on repeated sprint performance in men. J Strength Cond Res. 2003 Feb;17(1):47-52. Dunne L, Worley S, Macknin M. Ribose versus dextrose supplementation, association with rowing performance: a double-blind study. Clin J Sport Med. 2006 Jan;16(1):68-71.

Gallagher PM, Williamson DL, et al. Effects of ribose supplementation on adenine nucleotide concentration in skeletal muscle following high–intensity exercise. Midwest Regional Chapter of the ACSM, October (2000).

Gross M, Kormann B, Zollner N. Ribose administration during exercise: effects on substrates and products of energy metabolism in healthy subjects and a patient with myoadenylate deaminase deficiency. Klin Wochenschr. 1991 Feb 26;69(4):151-5.

Gross M, Gresser U. Ergometer exercise in myoadenylate deaminase deficient patients. Clin Investig. 1993 Jun;71(6):461-5.

Hellsten–Westing Y, Balsom PD, Norman B, Sjodin B. The effect of high–intensity training on purine metabolism in man. Acta Physiol Scand. 1993 Dec; 149(4):405-12.

Kreider RB, Melton C, Greenwood M, et al. Effects of oral D–ribose supplementation on anaerobic capacity and selected metabolic markers in healthy males. Int J Sport Nutr Exerc Metab. 2003 Mar;13(1):76-86.

Op 't Eijnde B, Van Leemputte M, Brouns F, et al. No effects of oral ribose supplementation on repeated maximal exercise and de novo ATP resynthesis. J Appl Physiol. 2001 Nov;91(5):2275-81.

Witter J , Gallagher P, et al. Effects of ribose supplementation on performance during repeated high–intensity cycle sprints. Midwest Regional Chapter of the ACSM, October (2000).

ȹ

Chapter 3

PROTEIN POWDERS

P rotein powders are among the most popular supplements on the market today. It isn't always easy or convenient to get the desired amount of protein from whole foods, so supplemental protein is used to fill in the blanks. All proteins are not alike, and some possess clear advantages over others, particularly at certain times. Certain combinations might also

Protien Powders Covered

❖ **Casein**

❖ **Colostrum**

❖ **Egg White Protein**

❖ **Serum Protein Isolate**

❖ **Vegetarian Proteins: Soy, Hemp, Rice**

❖ **Whey Protein**

have advantages, both for addition of LBM as well as basic health and well-being. It's important to remember that protein powders are supplements. In other words, you use them in addition to the food in your diet – not to replace food in your diet.

Protein powders typically supply very few additional nutrients besides protein. Far too many would be bodybuilders construct their diets around protein powders or other supplements, such as weight gainers and MRPs, then wonder why they're not seeing results. While isn't a hard and fast rule, I recommend that you consume no more than 30% of your total protein from supplements.

A fairly normal schedule might be something like: Breakfast, mid morning shake, lunch, post-workout shake, snack, dinner.

Used correctly, high quality protein powders are one of the best supplement investments you can make.

CASEIN

What is it?

Casein is the dominant type of protein in cow's milk, comprising 80% of the total. There are several different types of caseins: alpha(s1), alpha(s2), beta, and kappa. These associate together to form large, complex structures known as micelles. Casein micelles are huge and vary in size, but have an average molecular weight of 2.8 x 108.

What is it supposed to do?

Casein is used primarily as an anti-catabolic—that is, a protein to help limit muscle breakdown.

What does the research say for athletic performance?

Casein has been making inroads with athletes for a variety of reasons; some scientific in nature and some based on over–hyped marketing by supplement companies looking to sell an alternative to the over saturated whey market. Unlike whey, where there has been quite a bit of research showing the undenatured forms are the most biologically active, there is little research to show either form of casein is superior to the other, regarding effects on muscle mass or other issues that relate to athletes. People should not be overly swayed by ads from supplement companies claiming one form has been "proven" superior over another at this time.

Since many of the recent studies have used the micellar form—and it's logical to think the human body prefers the native form—we will assume for now (and assuming is a very dangerous thing to do in the world of science) that micellar casein is the superior form of casein. More research is clearly needed however.

One study in particular called "Slow and fast dietary proteins differently modu-late postprandial protein accretion" was responsible for causing a resurgence of interest in casein and led to a great deal of misinformation, disinformation, and downright fabrication, by supplement companies and pretend experts looking to either sell casein or bash it to protect their own sale of whey.

The truth behind the study that caused all the excitement was damn near impossible to find…until now. The basic premise of this much touted study was that the speed of absorption of dietary amino acids (from ingested proteins) varies according to the type of dietary protein a person eats. The researchers wanted to see if the type of protein eaten would affect postprandial (e.g., after a meal) protein synthesis, breakdown, and deposition. To test the hypothesis, They fed casein (CAS) and whey protein (WP) to a group of healthy adults who had been fasted.

Here is what they found:

- WP induced a dramatic but short increase of plasma amino acids.

- CAS induced a prolonged plateau of moderate increase in amino acids (hyperaminoacidemia)

- Whole body protein breakdown was inhibited by 34% after CAS ingestion but not after WP ingestion.

- Postprandial protein synthesis was stimulated by 68% with the WP meal and to a lesser extent (+31%) with the CAS meal.

There was of course far more detailed findings (relating mostly to postprandial whole body leucine oxidation rates, etc.) which I wont go into as it's not really needed for this section.

The researchers of this study concluded:

" …the speed of protein digestion and amino acid absorption from the gut has a major effect on whole body protein anabolism after one single meal…"

Basically the study found that CAS was good at preventing protein breakdown (proteolysis) but not so good for increasing protein synthesis and WP had basically the opposite effects: it increased protein synthesis but didn't prevent protein breakdown.

The reason for this is that whey is absorbed rapidly (being a highly soluble protein) and much of it is oxidized while casein forms a "clot" in the gut and is absorbed slowly (being a fairly insoluble protein), thus causing a steady level of amino acids. That's why they dubbed whey a "fast" protein and casein a "slow" protein.

So far so good right?

So what can we conclude from this study and how useful are the results? Like so many studies, the results were interesting and the results were of little use to people in the real world. Why? Because the subjects were fasted (had not eaten for a long period of time) which of course does not reflect how people—especially bodybuilders and other athletes—actually eat. Do these results hold up under more "real world" conditions where people are eating every few hours and/or mixing the proteins with other macro nutrients (i.e., carbs and fats)?

The answer is probably not, which is exactly what the same researchers found when they attempted to mimic a more realistic eating pattern. Their follow up study was called "The digestion rate of protein is an independent regulating factor of postprandial protein retention."

Four groups of five to six healthy young men received:

- A single meal of slowly digested casein (CAS).

- A single meal of free amino acid mimicking casein composition (AA).

- A single meal of rapidly digested whey proteins (WP).

- Or repeated meals of whey proteins (RPT–WP) mimicking slow digestion rate (i.e., reflecting how people really eat).

So what did they find?

In a nut shell, giving people multiple doses of whey—which mimics how people really eat—had basically the same effects as a single dose of casein, and mixing either with fats and proteins pretty much nullified any big differences between the two proteins. All I can say to that is (drum roll)…no duh! Their more technical conclusion was:

> "The fast meals induced a strong, rapid, and transient increase of aminoacidemia, leucine flux, and oxidation. After slow meals, these parameters increased moderately but durably. Postprandial leucine balance over 7 h was higher after the slow than after the fast meals (CAS: 38 +/– 13 vs. AA: –12 +/– 11, $P < 0.01$; RPT–WP: 87 +/– 25 vs. WP: 6 +/– 19 micromol/kg, $P < 0.05$). Protein digestion rate is an independent factor modulating postprandial protein deposition."

And even that is not the end of the story as multiple follow up studies done by the same group and others found that these effects could even be different in older versus younger people and male versus female! How messed up is that?!

OK, can we confuse the issue some more? Yup.

A study called "Effect of a hypocaloric diet, increased protein intake and resistance training on lean mass gains and fat mass loss in overweight police officers" found some interesting and seemingly conflicting results to the studies outlined above.

This study looked at the effects of a moderate hypocaloric (low calorie) high-protein diet and resistance training, using whey or casein, versus the diet alone on body composition. A randomized, prospective 12 week study was performed comparing the changes in body composition produced by three different treatment modalities in three study groups.

- One group (n = 10) was placed on a nonlipogenic, hypocaloric diet alone (80% of predicted needs).

-   A second group (n = 14) was placed on the hypocaloric diet plus resistance exercise plus a high-protein intake (1.5 g/kg/day) using a casein protein hydrolysate.

-   The third group (n = 14) treatment was identical to the second, except for the use of a whey protein hydrolysate.

The study found that weight loss was approximately the same in all three groups with each losing approximately 2.5 kgs. But if you look at it, the actual fat loss and changes in LBM between groups were quite different. The mean fat loss was 2.5, 7.0, and 4.2 kg in the three groups, respectively, so the casein group lost more fat. As expected, increases in LBM in the three groups did not change for diet alone, versus gains of 4 and 2 kg in the casein and whey groups, respectively.

Translated, the casein group lost more fat and added more LBM then the whey group or the non-supplemented non-exercising group. This translated into greater strength increases for the casein group then for the whey group (mean increase in strength for chest, shoulder and legs was approximately 59% for casein and approximately 29% for whey, a significant group to group difference). The researchers concluded:

"This significant difference in body composition and strength is likely due to improved nitrogen retention and overall anti-catabolic effects caused by the peptide components of the casein hydrolysate."

What about real world athletic performance?

Bodybuilders have taken to the idea of using casein as a "bedtime snack" to limit muscle protein breakdown during sleep. Many also use it—alone or combined with whey—for general protein supplementation during the day. Most seem to feel that it's a worthwhile addition, although it's impossible to assess what effect it has on adding LBM.

Will Brink's Recommendation

So where does all this leave us? From the research we have to go on and applying it to the real world, there are some basic conclusions we come to regarding casein and the issue of casein versus whey:

Nature combines the two for a reason as both proteins have some unique effects.

If one is eating as they should for increases in LBM as outlined prior, there is probably no effective differences between the two proteins.

Mixing the proteins with fats and carbs will also alter the effects on the rate of absorption.

Whey is probably superior post-workout when a fast absorption of protein is warranted.

Casein is probably best used when there will be prolonged periods of time without eating, in particular, during sleep. 30-50 g of casein before bed may have anti-catabolic benefits.

MRPs (i.e., products that attempt to replace a meal like Lean Body®, MetRX®, etc) are probably most effective when they combine whey and casein as nature does. Cow's milk is approximately 80% casein and 20% whey. Human mothers milk is closer to a 50/50 split, so anything between those two is probably optimal for a commercial or homemade MRP.

During reduced calories (e.g., diets for losing fat) casein may be the better protein for preventing a loss of LBM due to its slow absorption/anti-catabolic effects. Combing the two in a 80/20 to 50/50 split of casein to whey may be optimal (though more data is CLEARLY needed!).

In my view, whey can do so many things that casein simply can't do, so I would not recommend people switch from whey to casein exclusively. I would recommend that people consider using the two proteins strategically as outlined above. The benefits of the two proteins appear to be in the timing of both.

References

Boirie Y, Dangin M, Gachon P, et al. Slow and fast dietary proteins differently modulate postprandial protein accretion. Proc Natl Acad Sci U S A. 1997 Dec23;94(26):14930-5.

Dangin M, Boirie Y, Garcia–Rodenas C, et al. The digestion rate of protein is an independent regulating factor of postprandial protein retention. Am J Physiol Endocrinol Metab. 2001 Feb;280(2):E340-8.

Dangin M, Boirie Y, Guillet C, Beaufrere B. Influence of the protein digestion rate on protein turnover in young and elderly subjects. J Nutr. 2002 Oct;132(10):3228S-33S.

Dangin M, Guillet C, Garcia–Rodenas C, et al. The rate of protein digestion affects protein gain differently during aging in humans. J Physiol. 2003 Jun 1;549(Pt 2):635-44. Epub 2003 Mar 28.

Demling RH, DeSanti L. Effect of a hypocaloric diet, increased protein intake and resistance training on lean mass gains and fat mass loss in overweight police officers. Ann Nutr Metab. 2000;44(1):21-9.

φ

COLOSTRUM

What is it?

Colostrum—also called foremilk—is a thin, yellowish fluid secreted by the mammary glands of mammals in the very first week of lactation. It's rich in immunoglobulins, anti–microbial peptides, minerals and multitude of growth factors conferred to the infant (in humans) or calf (in cows and other animals).

What is it supposed to do?

Colostrum is rich in growth factors, including IGF–1. Some studies have shown colostrum supplements increase IGF–1, and have a positive influence on lean body mass and/or athletic performance.

What does the research say for athletic performance?

From a medical standpoint, properly made colostrum looks promising for diseases that affect the gastrointestinal (GI) tract. Several studies have confirmed colostrum's potential to protect against and treat GI infections. One study that found colostrum increased the salivary Insulin Like Growth Factor one (IGF–1) levels of athletes. Nine male sprinters were fed a colostrum product for 8 days.

The study found statistically significant changes in the IGF–1 levels of the athletes tested via saliva testing. At one point, it was thought that this result showed that the long–held belief that IGF–1 was degraded in the digestive tract might be wrong. A follow up study by the same research group, concluded:

" ...a long–term supplementation of bovine colostrum (Dynamic) increases serum IGF–I and saliva IgA concentration in athletes during training. Absorption data show that ingested 123I–rhIGF–I is fragmented in circulation and that no radioactive IGF–I is eluted

at the positions of free, or the IGF, binding proteins, giving no support to the absorption of IGF–I from bovine colostrum."

The researchers did find a 17% increase in serum IGF–1 with 20 g/day colostrum supplementation, but speculated the increase might be due to enhanced stimulation of IGF–1 synthesis.

The results from different studies of the effects of colostrum supplementation on lean body mass and performance are conflicting. One study presented by Dr. Richard Kreider and co–workers at the 2001 Experimental Biology conference found the addition of colostrum to the diets of 49 well trained athletes increased both body weight and bench press strength. A study conducted by Dr. Jose Antonio found a mean increase of 1.49 kg of lean body mass after 8 weeks of supplementing with 20 g/day colostrum. Small, but significant improvements in cycling, jumping and sprint performance have also been demonstrated.

On the other hand, 60 g/day colostrum did not improve the performance of elite female rowers, while 20 g/day had no effect on strength performance or net protein balance.

In addition, two of the studies that showed positive effects on performance showed no increases in serum IGF–1.

What about real world athletic performance?

I haven't heard much—either positive or negative—about colostrum supplementation. Very few people use it at the doses seen in the studies due to the expense; and the smaller doses found in capsule formulations are highly unlikely to have any significant effects on LBM or performance. Colostrum is included as an ingredient in several popular protein powders, but appears to be mostly label decoration.

Will Brink's Recommendation

Should athletes run out and buy colostrum? Possibly not. Some of the above studies were small; while most of the ones showing positive effects on performance resulted in fairly modest improvements. Conflicting results make it difficult to come to any firm conclusions.

Part of the problem may lie in the differences between products. There is no standard for the composition of colostrum, which can vary considerably based on the health of the cows, feed composition, collection times, and processing. Collection time is a significant issue: colostrum is defined as the milk collected up to 4 days following calving. Nonetheless, the colostrum collected within the first 24 hours is far richer in immunoglobulins than the colostrum collected at later intervals. This may also be true for other growth factors as well.

It appears that newer versions of colostrum may, in fact, have benefit to athletes and appear to have clear uses in certain medical conditions. How much benefit and at what dosage have yet to be determined. I think colostrum is worth keeping an eye on and maybe useful for various pathologies of the digestive tract. In my view, it might be worth a try just for the heck of it, although it's a fairly expensive supplement. Optimal doses are unknown at this time, although 20 g/day is the one most commonly seen in the studies, which gets expensive real fast…

References

Antonio J, Sanders MS, Van Gammeren D. The effects of bovine colostrum supplementation on body composition and exercise performance in active men and women. Nutrition. 2001 Mar;17(3):243-7.

Brinkworth GD, Buckley JD. Bovine colostrum supplementation does not affect plasma buffer capacity or haemoglobin content in elite female rowers. Eur J Appl Physiol. 2004 Mar;91(2-3):353-6.

Buckley JD, Brinkworth GD, Abbott MJ. Effect of bovine colostrum on anaerobic exercise performance and plasma insulin–like growth factor I. J Sports Sci. 2003 Jul;21(7):577-88.

Buckley JD, Abbott MJ, Brinkworth GD, Whyte PB. Bovine colostrum supplementation during endurance running training improves recovery, but not performance. J Sci Med Sport. 2002 Jun;5(2):65-79.

Coombes JS, Conacher M, Austen SK, Marshall PA. Dose effects of oral bovine colostrum on physical work capacity in cyclists. Med Sci Sports Exerc. 2002 Jul;34(7):1184-8.

Hofman Z, Smeets R, Verlaan G, et al. The effect of bovine colostrum supplementation on exercise performance in elite field hockey players. Int J Sport Nutr Exerc Metab. 2002 Dec;12(4):461-9.

Kelly GS. Bovine colostrums: a review of clinical uses.Altern Med Rev. 2003 Nov;8(4):378-94.

Mero A, Miikkulainen H, Riski J, et al. Effects of bovine colostrum supplementation on serum IGF–I, IgG, hormone, and saliva IgA during training. J Appl Physiol. 1997 Oct;83(4):1144-51.

Mero A, Nykanen T, Keinanen O, et al. Protein metabolism and strength performance after bovine colostrum supplementation. Amino Acids. 2005 May; 28(3):327-35. Epub 2005 Mar 25.

Playford RJ, Macdonald CE, Johnson WS. Colostrum and milk–derived peptide growth factors for the treatment of gastrointestinal disorders. Am J Clin Nutr. 2000Jul;72(1):5-14.

Shing CM, Jenkins DG, Stevenson L, Coombes JS. The influence of bovine colostrum supplementation on exercise performance in highly trained cyclists. Br J Sports Med. 2006 Sep;40(9):797-801.

EGG WHITE PROTEIN

What is it?

Eggs—in particular egg whites—have been a staple protein source for bodybuilders and other athletes for decades. Egg white, or albumen, is composed of several different proteins:

ovalbumin (54%)

conalbumin (13%)

ovomucoid (11%)

globulins (8%)

lysozyme (3.5%)

ovomucin (1.5%)

other proteins present at <1%: flavoprotein, ovoglycoprotein, ovomacroglobulin, ovoinhibitor and avidin

Supplemental egg white protein is sold as a spray-dried powder, or in liquid, pasteurized form.

What is it supposed to do?

Egg white protein is a virtually fat-free, low–calorie source of protein. While egg white proteins are not—as far as is currently known—a source of bioactive peptides (such as whey, etc.), they can be used to increase the overall protein content of the diet.

What does the research say for athletic performance?

Beyond serving as a source of protein, there is little that's special about egg whites. Substituting egg white protein in the diets of hypercholesterolemic women had beneficial effects on serum lipids. Egg white is also relatively high in BCAAs, so can be used in addition to other protein supplements such as whey as a source of these critical amino acids.

There is the myth pushed by various raw food devotees, that eating denatured proteins is somehow harmful and/or unhealthful. While most people wouldn't eat raw meat, they nonetheless will consume raw eggs, in the belief that cooking destroys the protein, or makes it less digestible.

But the precise opposite is true for egg whites. Research has shown that raw egg whites, in fact, are much more poorly absorbed than cooked ones. In two separate studies, raw egg whites consumed by human volunteers were 35%-50% undigested and absorbed, whereas only 5%-9% of cooked egg whites were not assimilated. The liquid egg whites sold refrigerated have been pasteurized. I've been asked if these whites are more digestible than fresh, raw whites. They probably are, but I doubt that they are as digestible as completely cooked whites.

What about real world athletic performance?

Many bodybuilders supplement their protein intake with egg whites; both cooked or blended with other proteins in a shake. It's a simple and convenient way to add extra protein, which is why it's such a common practice.

Will Brink's Recommendation

It should be emphasized that egg whites aren't good for much else besides protein. Most of the egg nutrients are contained in the yolk. So while egg whites can be used to boost the protein content of a meal, they shouldn't be used to replace more nutritious sources.

Another point of contention regarding egg whites is people are under the impression (often due to misleading marketing by companies selling egg white protein) that egg whites are some sort of super protein. It should be noted the high score eggs have is based on the whole egg only. For example, whole eggs score 100 on the biological value (BV) protein scoring system. Egg whites have a BV score of 88. While thats not a low quality protein per se, but it's not the BV of 100 whole eggs enjoy. Will this have any negative effects on your ability to gain LBM? Unlikely, but when ever you see companies calling their egg white protein product "natures perfect food" or "the gold standard protein" and other over hyped nonsense, remember it's whole eggs and not egg whites they are actually referring to.

References

Asato L, Wang MF, Chan YC, et al. Effect of egg white on serum cholesterol concentration in young women. J Nutr Sci Vitaminol (Tokyo). 1996 Apr;42(2):87-96.

Evenepoel P, Geypens B, Luypaerts A, et al. Digestibility of cooked and raw egg protein in humans as assessed by stable isotope techniques. J Nutr. 1998 Oct;128(10):1716-22.

Evenepoel P, Claus D, Geypens B, et al. Amount and fate of egg protein escaping assimilation in the small intestine of humans. Am J Physiol. 1999 Nov;277(5 Pt 1):G935-43.

φ

SERUM PROTEIN ISOLATE

What is it?

Serum protein isolate is one of the newer protein supplements to hit the market. It's derived from bovine blood serum or plasma. Plasma is the clear, straw–colored fluid remaining when the blood cells are removed—typically by centrifugation. Serum is the same, except the blood is allowed to clot before removing the fluid.

The major plasma proteins are: albumin, immunoglobulins (IgG, IgA, IgD, IgE, IgM), transferrin, and fibrinogen. There are also a large number of minor constituents: enzymes and various peptide and polypeptide growth factors, including IGF–1.

Serum protein isolate is being marketed primarily by Proliant, Inc. as "Immunolin." Proliant uses a proprietary manufacturing process, so the precise proportions of each component in Immunolin isn't public information.

Proliant also claims that Immunolin is BSE free. BSE is bovine spongiform encephalopathy, an infectious disease that causes progressive—and eventually fatal—neurodegeneration. Also known as "Mad Cow Disease", it can be passed to humans through contaminated meat and byproducts.

What is it supposed to do?

Proliant claims that the benefits of serum protein isolate are similar to those of colostrum. It's supposed to be a "value added" supplement that provides both high quality protein and immune enhancement.

What does the research say for athletic performance?

There is very little direct research on the value of serum/plasma protein in human nutrition. In one small study on the recovery of

10 Peruvian children suffering from severe protein-calorie malnutrition, bovine serum concentrate was used to replace either 25% or 50% of the milk protein in a control diet. The diet was well tolerated and no adverse effects were reported.

The lack of human data is balanced by a large number of animal feeding studies, most of which were conducted on weanling pigs. In nearly all of the studies reviewed, spray-dried plasma (either porcine or unspecified "animal" plasma) has been an effective feed amendment, that has had positive effects on both immune status and growth.

In one study, piglets weaned at 21 days of age were fed a diet containing 6% spray-dried animal plasma had improved growth and reduced inflammation following a challenge with enterotoxigenic E. coli K88. Similar effects were also seen in a study on the performance of early (10 day) weaned piglets challenged with E. coli strain F18.

Studies conducted in the absence of an immunological challenge have shown that adding spray-dried plasma to piglet feed increases weight gain and nitrogen retention. Most of these studies agree that the increase in growth is due primarily to increased feed intake: piglets display a clear preference for plasma-enriched feed. Furthermore, in one Proliant sponsored study, the actual percentage of fat vs. fat-free tissue was unchanged vs. controls. Thus plasma feeding leads to bigger, but not necessarily leaner, pigs. Researchers have also noted that supplemental methionine is needed when the plasma content of the diet exceeds 6%.

Spray-dried plasma contains a number of growth factors, including IGF–1. The piglet studies demonstrate that consuming spray-dried plasma does not increase levels of plasma IGF–1. This is in accord with a study demonstrating that oral IGF–1 in humans is broken down in the digestive tract.

This does not exclude the possibility of local effects of IGF–1 in the gut. There are IGF–1 receptors in the small intestine, and it's thought that IGF–1 along other growth factors such as EGF (epidermal growth factor) and TGF–a/TGF–b (transforming growth factor) play a role in the development of the small intestine in breast-fed human infants. There is no indication at the moment that this leads to skeletal muscle growth.

Several studies have demonstrated that oral administration of hyperimmune globulin (i.e., immunoglobulin preparations from specifically immunized animals) is a useful therapy for gastrointestinal infections, such as rotavirus and shigella. So it's possible that consumption of non-denatured immunoglobulins in bovine serum protein could have a protective effect against certain GI infections. This hasn't been demonstrated for Immunolin, however. It's also possible that the effects of consuming bovine serum protein will be similar to colostrum, although this hasn't been proven either.

What about real world athletic performance?

Immunolin is a fairly new supplement, and isn't cheap. There are at least a dozen brands using it on the market now, although most of them are protein blends. In general, the feedback I've seen on these products is good, although in line with most other well made protein powders that don't contain Immunolin.

Many users are a bit surprised to find out that what they are actually eating is spray dried blood!

Will Brink's Recommendation

Some of the ads I've seen for bovine serum protein claim that it's the "first protein to out–date whey protein." Needless to state, there's no data to support such a claim. There's very little information to support any improvements in lean mass, body composition or performance vs. whey or any other protein source, for that matter. Until there are some solid head-to-head studies on this new supplement vs. whey, the companies selling this stuff with claims of it being superior to whey, are blowing hot marketing air. The companies selling it are also going to great lengths to disguise the source of its production: cow's blood.

Though very unscientific of me, I find this product has a high yuk factor but that's just me…

I'd put this protein in the same category as colostrum: perhaps worth a try, although it's far from clear that the benefits are worth the extra price.

References

Cummins AG, Thompson FM. Effect of breast milk and weaning on epithelial growth of the small intestine in humans. Gut. 2002 Nov;51(5):748-54.

de Rodas BZ, Sohn KS, Maxwell CV, Spicer LJ. et al. Plasma protein for pigs weaned at 19 to 24 days of age: effect on performance and plasma insulin–like growth factor I, growth hormone, insulin, and glucose concentrations. J Anim Sci. 1995 Dec;73(12):3657-65.

Grinstead GS, Goodband RD, Dritz SS, et al. Effects of a whey protein product and spray-dried animal plasma on growth performance of weanling pigs. J Anim Sci. 2000 Mar;78(3):647-57.

Jiang R, Chang X, Stoll B, et al. Dietary plasma protein is used more efficiently than extruded soy protein for lean tissue growth in early–weaned pigs. J Nutr. 2000 Aug;130(8):2016-9.

Jiang R, Chang X, Stoll B, et al. Dietary plasma protein reduces small intestinal growth and lamina propria cell density in early weaned pigs. J Nutr. 2000 Jan;130(1):21-6.

Kats LJ, Nelssen JL, Tokach MD, et al. The effect of spray-dried porcine plasma on growth performance in the early–weaned pig. J Anim Sci. 1994 Aug; 72(8):2075-81.

Sarker SA, Casswall TH, Mahalanabis D, et al. Successful treatment of rotavirus diarrhea in children with immunoglobulin from immunized bovine colostrum. Pediatr Infect Dis J. 1998 Dec;17(12):1149-54.

Tacket CO, Binion SB, Bostwick E, et al. Efficacy of bovine milk immunoglobulin concentrate in preventing illness after Shigella flexneri challenge. Am J Trop Med Hyg. 1992 Sep;47(3):276-83.

Thomson JE, Jones EE, Eisen EJ. Effects of spray-dried porcine plasma protein on growth traits and nitrogen and energy balance in mice. J Anim Sci. 1995 Aug;73(8):2340-6.

ቀ

VEGETARIAN PROTEINS: SOY, HEMP, RICE

What are they?

Soy protein isolate, hemp protein, and brown rice protein concentrate are all plant-based protein powders.

What are they supposed to do?

People who are vegans or have allergies to milk and/or egg proteins prefer these protein supplements. Soy protein is also marketed heavily to women, due to its phytoestrogen content.

What does the research say for athletic performance?

1. *Soy Protein Isolate*

The pluses and minuses of soy protein are covered in detail in my article, "The (Partial) Vindication of Soy Protein" on the Brinkzone, Read "The (Partial) Vindication of Soy Protein:

In brief, soy protein isolates have some interesting benefits; soy has been shown to reduce cholesterol, improve cardiovascular health and possibly increase thyroid output. In addition to the above benefits, more recent research has shown that soy protein intake can increase antioxidant levels and reduce oxidation of LDL–cholesterol.

The drawbacks are equally well known. The biggest one is that soy protein has a lower biological value than animal proteins such as whey or egg. Proponents of soy protein frequently point to a newer measure of protein quality: the PDCAAS (Protein Digestibility Corrected Amino Acid Score), and insist that soy rates just as high as these animal proteins—all have the same, perfect 1.00 (100%) rating. What they neglect to mention, however, is that the PDCAAS—which is used by the World Health Organization for rating the adequacy of protein sources for malnourished children in developing countries—is arbitrarily cut off at 1.00.

Whey and egg proteins actually score higher, but the excess is not reported. The actual PDCAAS for whey is 1.14, whereas the best score I've seen reported for a soy protein isolate is a true 1.00. I would never argue that high quality, methionine–fortified isolates aren't adequate for enriching the diets of malnourished children, or are otherwise inadequate for basic growth and development...but I would argue that they're suboptimal compared to a protein like whey for supplementing a bodybuilding diet.

2. *Hemp Protein*

Hemp is the common term for Cannabis sativa, also known as marijuana. But long before it was used to get high, Cannabis was a source of both fiber for fabric and rope, as well as oil seeds for food. The hemp currently being cultivated has been bred to have a negligible amount of the psychoactive compound THC found in marijuana.

Hemp seeds are quite nutritious. Hemp seeds are 34.6% protein, and 46.5% fat. They are high in fiber and contain the omega–3 essential fatty acid alpha–linolenic acid, along with the omega–6 gamma–linolenic acid.

The hemp protein currently sold in health food stores is derived from the seed cake left over after pressing the oil. The protein contains about 35%-45% protein, along with a residual amount of oil. The protein is also high in chlorophyll and other nutrients associated with the seeds (vitamin E, magnesium and zinc).

There are very few studies on the consumption of hemp foods. One feeding study on hens showed no adverse effects on egg production, feed consumption, feed efficiency, body weight change or egg quality. Human studies have been confined to evaluating whether or not consumption of hemp foods could result in false positive drug tests (they don't).

On the negative side, it's unlike other protein powders: it's not highly processed or refined, so has a gritty, grassy taste. Due to the oil content, it also needs to be kept refrigerated.

3. *Brown Rice Protein Concentrate*

Brown rice protein concentrate is a non-allergenic alternative to soy protein isolate. Oryzatein™ is a version recently introduced to the market. According to the manufacturer, Axiom Foods, Oryzatein™ has an absorption ratio (AR) of 98.6%, a, biological value (BV) of 77%, a Protein Efficiency Ratio (PER) of 2.75, a Protein Digestibility–Corrected Amino Acid Scoring (PDCAAS) of 1.00, and a net protein utilization (NPU) of 75.92 in growing rats. If true, it's at least equivalent to, and perhaps a bit better than soy protein.

The company also claims that Oryzatein™ has an amino acid profile "...with an approx. 98% correlation to mother's milk and an approx. 97% correlation to whey." Since the actual amino acid profile of the product has not been made available, the truth of this claim remains to be seen. There are other concentrates on the market that range from 50–80% protein.

Feeding studies on rice protein concentrate are also limited. One study in piglets rated rice protein concentrate favorably as a protein source. It did not score as high in amino acid or ileal digestion as the animal protein sources tested (whey protein concentrate, spray-dried plasma, and salmon protein hydrolysate), but still gave good results.

What about real world athletic performance?

For vegans or people with milk or egg protein allergies, soy, hemp and rice proteins offer alternatives that most users appear to be happy with. Many non-vegetarians also find that supplementing with plant proteins (esp. soy and hemp) have health uses beyond the addition of protein.

Will Brink's Recommendation

Supplementing with some soy protein isolate can be useful, even for non-vegetarian bodybuilders. And, as long as you don't mind the taste/texture/color, hemp protein can also provide some benefits. Rice protein appears to be a decent alternative for people with allergies to milk or soy (though its bad for those who may have a rice allergy!) who want to use a protein supplement.

But unless you are a vegan, or have health or ethical issues that restrict the use of milk or egg proteins, I would not substitute any of these for much more anabolic animal proteins.

References

Gottlob RO, DeRouchey JM, Tokach MD, et al. Amino acid and energy digestibility of protein sources for growing pigs. J Anim Sci. 2006 Jun;84(6):1396-402.

Janow, DJ. Oryzatein™, a novel brown rice protein that may be used as a hypoallergenic replacement for soy, whey, and casein proteins currently used in any food applications. 2005 IFT Annual Meeting, July 15-20 (Abstract).

Leson G, Pless P, Grotenhermen F, et al. Evaluating the impact of hemp food consumption on workplace drug tests. J Anal Toxicol. 2001 Nov-Dec; Chapter 5/Vegetarian Proteins 25(8):691-8.

Mahn K, Borras C, Knock GA, et al. Dietary soy isoflavone induced increases in antioxidant and eNOS gene expression lead to improved endothelial function and reduced blood pressure in vivo. FASEB J. 2005 Oct;19(12):1755-7.

Silversides FG, Lefrancois MR. The effect of feeding hemp seed meal to laying hens. Br Poult Sci. 2005 Apr;46(2):231-5.

ϕ

Whey Protein

What is it?

Whey protein in particular has become a staple supplement for most bodybuilders and other athletes and for good reason: it's a great protein for a wide variety of reasons. Whey proteins make up approx. 20% of the protein in milk. Whey protein is actually a mixture of proteins with different biological properties.

They are:

Beta–lactoglobulin (approx. 50%)

Alpha–lactalbumin (approx. 25%)

Bovine Serum Albumin

Immunoglobulins (antibodies): IgG1, IgG2, IgA, IgM

Glycomacropeptides

Lactoferrin

Lactoperoxidase

Lysozyme

Beta2–microglobulin

What is it supposed to do?

Whey protein is an extremely high quality source of essential amino acids that are easily digested and absorbed. But beyond its value as a source of dietary protein, it possesses a variety of potential health benefits. A growing number of studies have found that whey may potentially reduce cancer rates, combat HIV, improve immunity, reduce stress and lower cortisol, increase brain serotonin levels, improve liver function in those suffering from certain forms of hepatitis, reduce blood pressure, and improve performance, to name a few of its potential medical and sports related applications.

What does the research say for athletic performance?

One of whey's major effects is its apparent ability to raise glutathione (GSH). The importance of GSH for the proper function of the immune system cannot be overstated. GSH is arguably the most important water-soluble antioxidant found in the body. The concentration of intracellular GSH is directly related to lymphocytes reactivity to a challenge, which suggests intracellular GSH levels are one way to modulate immune function. GSH is a tri-peptide made up of the amino acids L–cysteine, L–glutamine and glycine. Of the three, cysteine is the main source of the free sulfhydryl group of GSH and is a limiting factor in the synthesis of GSH.

Since GSH is known to be essential to immunity, oxidative stress, general well-being, and reduced levels of GSH are associated with a long list of diseases, whey has a place in anyone's nutrition program. Reduced GSH is also associated with over training syndrome (OTS) in athletes, so whey may very well have an application in preventing, or at least mitigating, OTS. As mentioned previously, GSH is the major intracellular water-soluble antioxidant in the body, which is involved in the recycling of other antioxidants.

Twenty healthy young adults (10 men, 10 women) were supplemented with either whey or casein for 3 months. The researchers looked at:

- Muscular performance (as assessed by whole leg isokinetic cycle testing)
- Lymphocyte GSH levels (as a marker of tissue GSH).

As one would expect, they found no baseline differences in peak power or work capacity between the whey and casein groups. However, after treatment, a follow up study on 18 subjects—9 who received the whey and 9 who received the casein (considered a placebo in this study) —was conducted.

Both peak power and work capacity increased significantly in the whey group, with no changes found in the casein group. Lymphocyte GSH also increased by over 35 percent in the group receiving the whey with no change in the group getting casein. The researchers concluded:

" This is the first study to demonstrate that prolonged supplementation with a product designed to augment antioxidant defenses resulted in improved volitional performance"

As mentioned, due to whey's high biological value and its other properties, such as a high branched chain amino acid content, etc., it has always been theorized whey should be a particularly effective protein for gaining or preserving muscle mass. This is one reason whey is the best selling protein on the market with bodybuilders.

A number of studies have now been performed that have confirmed what we already know: that whey protein—taken at the right time—can enhance lean body mass and performance.

For example, a study performed by Burke et al (2001) showed that consumption of whey protein with or without creatine, was associated with greater gains in lean mass and performance relative to controls. Tipton et al. (2004) demonstrated that whey, consumed either before or after resistance training, stimulated a positive anabolic response. Borsheim et al (2004) found that a post-workout drink of whey, carbohydrates and amino acids stimulated muscle protein synthesis to a greater extent than carbohydrate alone. Koopman et al (2005) had similar results using a post-workout beverage composed of whey protein hydrolysate, carbohydrate and leucine.

Another study by Chromiak et al (2004) demonstrated greater gains in lean body mass with a post-workout recovery drink containing whey protein, amino acids, creatine and carbohydrate vs. carbohydrate alone.

Several other studies have also shown the value of pre– and/or post-workout consumption of whey combined with casein. Kerksick et al (2006) found the greatest gains in lean mass using combination of 40 g/day whey protein + 8 g/day casein, while Hulmi et al (2005) demonstrated that consuming 25 g of combined whey and casein before training significantly increased post-workout metabolic rate.

What about real world athletic performance?

Many people have found whey protein to be a useful addition to their diets. Part of the reason for this is that whey protein products have evolved over the years and are far superior to other protein supplements due to the range of biologically active fractions now available.

When we talk about whey, we are actually referring to a complex protein made up of many smaller protein subfractions such as: beta–lactoglobulin, alpha–lactalbumin, immunoglobulins (IgGs), glycomacropeptides, bovine serum albumin (BSA), as well as minor constituents, such as lactoperoxidases, lysozyme and lactoferrin.

Each of the subfractions found in whey has its own unique biological properties. Up until quite recently, separating these subfractions on a large scale was either impossible or prohibitively expensive for anything but research purposes. Modern filtering technology has improved dramatically in the past decade, allowing companies to separate some of the highly bioactive peptides from whey, such as lactoferrin and lactoperoxidase.

Many of these subfractions are only found in very minute amounts in cow's milk, normally at less than one percent. For example, though one of the most promising subfractions for preventing various diseases, improving immunity and overall health, lactoferrin makes up approximately 0.5-1 percent or less of whey protein derived from cow's milk (whereas human milk contains up to 15 percent lactoferrin).

Over the past few decades, whey protein powders have evolved through several generations. The early whey protein products contained as little as 30-40 percent protein and had high amounts of lactose, fat, and denatured proteins. They were considered "concentrates" and were used mostly by the food industry for baking and other uses.

Many whey products sold today would be considered second–generation whey protein supplements. Most second-generation formulas are a mix of whey concentrates (WPC) and whey isolates (WPIs). WPCs now contain as high as 70-80 percent protein, with small amounts of lactose and fat. They generally contain as much as 90-96 percent undenatured proteins. Research has found that only whey proteins in their natural, undenatured state (i.e. native conformation) have biological activity. Processing whey protein to remove the lactose, fats, etc., without losing its biological activity, takes special care by the manufacturer. The protein must be processed under low temperature and/or low acid conditions as not to "denature" the protein.

Maintaining the natural undenatured state of the proteins is essential to whey's anti-cancer and immune stimulating activity. Most second-generation whey products are mixed with an isolate (WPI) to bring up the protein content per serving. WPIs contain >90 percent protein contents with minimal lactose and virtually no fat. Many isolates sold that are touted by supplement companies, are ion exchange isolates. This isolate is made by taking a concentrate and running it through what is called an "ion exchange" column. Proteins are selectively bound, based on their charge, while other components are removed.

Sounds pretty fancy, but there are serious drawbacks to this method. As mentioned above, whey protein is a complex mixture of different proteins that have their own unique effects on health, immunity, etc. Some of these subfractions are only found in very small amounts.

Due to the nature of the ion exchange process, the most valuable and health promoting components are selectively depleted. Though the protein content is increased, many of the most important subfractions are lost or greatly reduced. This makes ion exchange isolates a poor choice for a true third-generation whey protein supplement, though many companies still use it as their isolate source.

With the array of more recent processing techniques used to make WPI's—or pull out various subfractions—such as such ultra filtration (UF), micro filtration (MF), reverse osmosis (RO), dynamic membrane filtration (DMF), ion exchange chromatography, (IEC), electro-ultrafiltration (EU), radial flow chromatography (RFC) and nano filtration (NF), manufacturers can now make what appears to be optimal WPI's for health and disease prevention.

Low temperature microfiltration techniques now allow for the production of very high protein contents (>90 percent), the retention of important subfractions, extremely low fat and lactose contents, and virtually no denatured proteins. As you would expect, these WPIs are more expensive than WPCs or ion exchange isolates. Another fairly new development is the ability to isolate certain bioactive subfractions on a large scale from whey proteins, such as lactoferrin or glycomacropeptide.

This was not possible to do on a large scale just a few years ago, but can be done today with modern filtering techniques employed by a small number of companies. This allows for a truly tailored protein supplement; manufacturers now have the ability to add back certain subfractions in amounts that can't be found in nature.

Take, for example, the subfraction lactoferrin. In many whey products, it is nonexistent due to the type of processing employed. Even the best whey products contain less than 1 percent lactoferrin, and more like 0.5 percent, of this small,but important microfraction. Some companies are now able to add extra back in, to get a true "designer" protein.

Whey also has an exceptionally high biological value rating (though sellers of whey make FAR too big a deal of that fact) and an exceptionally high BCAA content (see BCAA section for more information).

Will Brink's Recommendation

It should be clearly noted, that even if additional research does find that whey plays a direct role in helping athletes add muscle, no one has ever exploded with new muscle from the simple addition of whey to their diet, regardless of what some supplement companies would have you believe.

With that in mind, for general health and well-being, whey gets a big thumbs up. For potential effects on muscle mass and performance, it gets a (very) tentative thumbs up at this time.

References

Baruchel S, Viau G. In vitro selective modulation of cellular glutathione by a humanized native milk protein isolate in normal cells and rat mammary carcinoma model. Anticancer Res. 1996 May-Jun;16(3A):1095-9.

Borsheim E, Aarsland A, Wolfe RR. Effect of an amino acid, protein, and carbohydrate mixture on net muscle protein balance after resistance exercise.Int J Sport Nutr Exerc Metab. 2004 Jun;14(3):255-71.

Bounous, G., et al. Effect of supplementation with a cysteine donor on muscular performance. J App Phys. 1999 87(4):1381-5.

Bounous G, Molson J. Competition for glutathione precursors between the immune system and the skeletal muscle: pathogenesis of chronic fatigue syndrome. Med Hypotheses. 1999 Oct;53(4):347-9.

Bounous G, Papenburg R, Kongshavn PA, et al. Dietary whey protein inhibits the development of dimethylhydrazine induced malignancy. Clin Invest Med. 1988 Jun;11(3):213-7.

Bounous G, Kongshavn PA, Gold P. The immunoenhancing property of dietary whey protein concentrate. Clin Invest Med. 1988 Aug;11(4):271-8.

Burke DG, Chilibeck PD, Davidson KS, et al. The effect of whey protein supplementation with and without creatine monohydrate combined with resistance training on lean tissue mass and muscle strength. Int J Sport Nutr Exerc Metab. 2001 Sep;11(3):349-64.

Chromiak JA, Smedley B, Carpenter W, et al. Effect of a 10–week strength training program and recovery drink on body composition, muscular strength and endurance, and anaerobic power and capacity. Nutrition. 2004 May; 20(5):420-7.

Hulmi JJ, Volek JS, Selanne H, Mero AA. Protein ingestion prior to strength exercise affects blood hormones and metabolism. Med Sci Sports Exerc. 2005 Nov;37(11):1990-7.

Kennedy RS, Konok GP, Bounous G, et al. The use of a whey protein concentrate in the treatment of patients with metastatic carcinoma: a phase I–II clinical study. Anticancer Res. 1995 Nov–Dec;15(6B):2643-9.

Kerksick CM, Rasmussen CJ, Lancaster SL, et al. The effects of protein and amino acid supplementation on performance and training adaptations during ten weeks of resistance training. J Strength Cond Res. 2006 Aug;20(3):643-53.

Koopman R, Wagenmakers AJ, Manders RJ, et al. Combined ingestion of protein and free leucine with carbohydrate increases postexercise muscle protein synthesis in vivo in male subjects. Am J Physiol Endocrinol Metab. 2005 Apr;288(4):E645-53.

Kotler DP, Tierney AR, Wang J, Pierson RN Jr. Magnitude of body–cell–mass depletion and the timing of death from wasting in AIDS. Am J Clin Nutr. 1989 Sep;50(3):444-7.

Markus CR, Olivier B, de Haan EH. Whey protein rich in alpha–lactalbumin increases the ratio of plasma tryptophan to the sum of the other large neutral amino acids and improves cognitive performance in stress–vulnerable subjects. Am J Clin Nutr. 2002 Jun;75(6):1051-6.

McIntosh GH, Regester GO, Le Leu RK, et al. Dairy proteins protect against dimethylhydrazine–induced intestinal cancers in rats. J Nutr. 1995 Apr; 125(4):809-16.

Micke P, Beeh KM, Buhl R. Effects of long–term supplementation with whey proteins on plasma glutathione levels of HIV–infected patients. Eur J Nutr. 2002 Feb;41(1):12-8.

Sternhagen LG, Allen JC. Growth rates of a human colon adenocarcinoma cell line are regulated by the milk protein alpha–lactalbumin. Adv Exp Med Biol. 2001;501:115-20.

Tipton KD, Elliott TA, Cree MG, et al. Ingestion of casein and whey proteins result in muscle anabolism after resistance exercise. Med Sci Sports Exerc. 2004 Dec;36(12):2073-81.

Tsai WY, Chang WH, Chen CH, Lu FJ. Enchancing effect of patented whey protein isolate (Immunocal) on cytotoxicity of an anticancer drug. Nutr Cancer. 2000;38(2):200-8.

Watanabe A, Okada K, Shimizu Y, et al. Nutritional therapy of chronic hepatitis by whey protein (non-heated). J Med. 2000;31(5–6):283-302.

ቇ

Chapter

4

ESSENTIAL ELEMENTS

E ssential elements are nutrients we need to get in our diet; vitamins, minerals and essential fatty acids. Vitamins are organic compounds that play a wide variety of important roles in metabolism. The most important role vitamins play is as co–factors for various enzyme reactions. Most of the compounds identified as vitamins need to be obtained from food—our bodies cannot

Essential Elements Covered
❖ Calcium
❖ Chromium Picolinate
❖ Essential Fatty Acids
❖ Fish Oil
❖ Vanadyl Sulfate
❖ Vitamin C
❖ Vitamin E
❖ ZMA

synthesize them. A failure to obtain adequate amounts of one or more vitamins results in deficiency diseases.

Several well known deficiency diseases include Scurvy (deficiency of vitamin C) and Beriberi (deficiency of thiamin—or vitamin B1).

Vitamins are classified as either water soluble or fat soluble. In general, water-soluble vitamins are readily excreted, so it's hard to consume toxic amounts. Fat-soluble vitamins, on the other hand, can be stored in the body, and long term and over consumption of certain ones (e.g., vitamin A and vitamin D) can lead to symptoms of toxicity.

There are 13 vitamins that are considered to be essential to human nutrition:

thiamin (B1)	folic acid
riboflavin (B2)	retinol/retinal/retinoic acid (vitamin A)
niacin/niacinamide (B3)	ascorbic acid (vitamin C)
pantothenic acid (B5)	Calcitriol (the active form of vitamin D)
pyridoxal/pyridoxamine/ pyridoxine (B6)	tocopherols/tocotrienols (members of the vitamin E family)
cobalamin (B12)	menaquinone (the active form of vitamin K)
biotin	

Minerals likewise perform essential functions. These are subdivided into two groups: major minerals and trace minerals.

Major minerals are:	Trace minerals are:
Calcium	Chromium
Chloride	Copper
Magnesium	Fluoride
Phosphorus	Iodine
Potassium	Iron
Sodium	Manganese
Sulfur	Molybdenum
	Selenium
	Zinc

Major minerals are required in amounts greater than 100 mg/ day. We need less of the trace minerals—some are needed in only microgram amounts (1 mcg = one-millionth of a gram).

To write about each of these would make for a very long (and quite boring) book! So for the sake of time and space I will only touch on the ones that are of particular interest to athletes, as well as a couple of other mineral products; ZMA and Vanadyl Sulfate.

Essential fatty acids have already been touched on in with more details to follow in this chapter.

CALCIUM

What is it?

Calcium is an essential mineral found in dairy foods, certain vegetables, tofu and in functional foods such as orange juice. There are also a variety of calcium supplements available. The most common supplemental forms are calcium carbonate, calcium phosphate, and calcium citrate.

What is it supposed to do?

As most people are well aware, calcium is a mineral needed for healthy strong bones. What many people may be unaware of is calcium's essential role in hundreds of other bodily processes from nerve transmission to enzyme activation and the functioning of muscle tissue.

Calcium works in conjunction with other minerals such as potassium and sodium to allow muscles to contract as well as keep blood in the proper pH. Without calcium, you would not even be able to lift your head up much less lift a weight.

What does the research say for athletic performance?

Special pumps change the concentration of calcium, sodium, and potassium ions (known as Ca2+, Na+, and K+ respectively) in different compartments of muscle tissue to make it contract (generate force) and relax. To get slightly technical: at the level of the muscle cell, ATP is used up quickly in an attempt to satisfy energy requirements. As by-products of exercise build up, the delicate balance between Na+/K+, Ca2+ is disturbed, it is believed, resulting in fatigue. Ionic regulation is critical to muscle contraction and metabolism, needed for optimal muscle function during exercise.

Training enhances K+ regulation in muscle and blood and reduces the rate of fatigue. Both endurance and strength training induces an increased muscle Na+,K+ pump concentration, usually associated with a reduced rise in plasma [K+] during exercise. Although impaired muscle Ca2+ regulation plays a vital role in fatigue, less is known about its actual effects on training.

Ok, enough technical talk.

There are other things that take place both inside and outside the muscle that add to fatigue, but that's for another place and time as the explanation would be...overly detailed. Interestingly, it has been found that athletes increase their rate of calcium loss in sweat from prolonged endurance sports, and increase their loss in urine after intense weight training.

There is some evidence to suggest that dairy calcium may be useful for helping to lose excess fat, but this has been questioned by other studies.

What about real world athletic performance?

I have yet to see anyone who added muscle, enhanced their strength, or improved their body composition simply by increasing their intake of calcium.

Will Brink's Recommendation

It's well established that most Americans fail to get even minimum intakes of calcium in their diet. Most athletes should be getting at least 1000 mg per day of calcium from food and/or supplemental sources, with female athletes needing even more.

Athletes should attempt to pay special attention to their calcium intakes and make sure to eat foods such as dairy products, leafy greens, cabbage, legumes and dairy based protein supplements. For example, there are many forms of well made whey proteins (i.e. concentrates, isolates, ion exchange, etc) that contain high amounts of calcium.

One 20 g scoop of whey can have as much as 120-150 mg of highly bioavailable calcium per serving. Micellar casein/caseinates are also a good source and can provide a third of the DRI (daily recommended intake) per scoop. Calcium gets a thumbs up for general health and possibly performance, but no solid data exists showing calcium has ergogenic effects above and beyond amounts needed for general health.

References

Green HJ. Mechanisms of muscle fatigue in intense exercise. J Sports Sci. 1997 Jun;15(3):247-56.

Lunde PK Verburg E, et al. Skeletal muscle fatigue in normal subjects and heart failure patients. Is there a common mechanism? Acta Physiol Scand. 1998 Mar;162(3):215-28.

Williams, M. Dietary supplements and sports performance: minerals. J Int Soc Sports Nutr. 2005; Feb;2(1):43-49.

ϙ

CHROMIUM PICOLINATE

What is it?

Chromium is a trace mineral that's essential for human health. Picolinic acid is an isomer of nicotinic acid (niacin) and is a chelating agent that enhances bioavailability.

What is it supposed to do?

Chromium picolinate is often found in OTC diet supplements as an aid to reduce body fat. Some writers also insist that it can increase muscle mass and athletic performance.

What does the research say for athletic performance?

Of all the nutrients that are sold for weight loss and increases in muscle mass, I can't think of a nutrient that has had a rockier track record in the research than chromium picolinate (CP).

Traditionally, sellers of CP tend to pay attention only to the research that showed this popular supplement could help with fat loss while increasing lean body mass (LBM).

The truth be known (which is the purpose of this section!), CP has had quite a checkered past as it relates to the effects of CP on body fat, muscle mass, and performance in different groups of people. Early research gave glowing reports of CP and showed significant reductions in body fat, with increases in muscle in college age athletes given CP supplements.

As recently as 1987, no less than six studies showed CP supplementation—using various populations of people ranging from the old to the young who took various doses of CP—found no effects on muscle mass or body fat.

In fact, one study found that older women (age range 54-71) given high doses of CP and put on a strength training regimen gained less muscle than the group that did not receive the supplement! On the flip side, a more recent study looks very promising for CP as a weight loss aid. A double blind placebo controlled study of 122 over weight people, given 400 mcg of CP for 90 days, lost over six pounds of body fat which was almost twice what the placebo group lost in body fat.

What about real world athletic performance?

Chromium picolinate is one of those supplements that look good on paper, but has been unimpressive in the real world. I have not seen anyone lose weight or improve their body composition due to the simple addition of chromium to their diet.

Will Brink's Recommendation

So how do we come to grips with all the conflicting research on chromium picolinate as a product used for weight loss and increase in muscle? It is well known that diets high in sugar, exercise and other factors drain the body's stores of chromium. It is also fairly well established that a large proportion of Americans do not take in sufficient amounts of chromium in their diets and we know that much of the foods people eat have been stripped of their chromium due to modern processing techniques.

Understandably, some research shows that a large proportion of people are chromium deficient. Finally, it is well established that chromium is an essential nutrient to human health and is critical for the regulation of proper blood sugar metabolism.

So, chromium is a nutrient that we should strive to get from a good supplement and from our food. For there is no doubt that people deficient in chromium will get positive effects from consuming more of it. Whether people who are not deficient in chromium will get any effect from additional chromium is questionable. So, make sure to get sufficient chromium in your diet from a variety of sources (i.e., multivitamins, whole grains, etc.), remembering, that to view any chromium supplement as a miracle fat loss supplement or muscle building/ergogenic sports aid would be premature at best.

For general health, CP gets a thumbs up, but for gaining muscle or increasing performance, it gets a thumbs down.

References

Preuss HG, Anderson RA. Chromium update: examining recent literature 1997-1998. Curr Opin Clin Nutr Metab Care. 1998 Nov;1(6):509-12.

Williams, M. Dietary supplements and sports performance: minerals. J Int Soc Sports Nutr. 2005; Feb;2(1):43-49.

ቅ

ESSENTIAL FATTY ACIDS: INCLUDES FLAX, FISH AND OTHERS

What are they?

As discussed in Chapter 1, the two essential fatty acids we need in our diets are linoleic acid (LA) which is an omega–6 fatty acid and alpha–linolenic acid (ALA) which is an omega–3 fatty acid. The highest known source of the omega–3 fatty acid ALA is flax oil which also contains a small amount of LA (flax oil has 4 :1 ratio of ALA to LA). Minimum requirements for essential fatty acids are 3–6% of daily calories for LA and 0.5-1% of daily calories for ALA.

What are they supposed to do?

Fish oils are well publicized omega–3 fatty acids that have been shown to have many benefits. From a general health standpoint, EFAs are involved in literally thousands of bodily processes essential to our health and general well-being: immunity, aging, hormone production and hormone signaling... well, you get the point.

As one would expect, EFAs have been found to have many health uses including cholesterol reduction, cancer treatment and prevention and treating inflammatory conditions.

In particular, the omega–3 fatty acids are anti–lipogenic (they block fat storage), anti-catabolic, anti-inflammatory, and they increase beta–oxidation (fat burning!), improve insulin sensitivity, increase thermogenesis, and have a whole lot more positive effects on fat loss that we don't have the space, time, or need, to cover in this little review.

Recent research has found that EFAs, in particular the omega–3 lipids, control gene transcription. For the more technically adept: omega–3 lipids play essential roles in the maintenance of energy balance and function as fuel partitioners in that they direct glucose toward glycogen storage, and direct fatty acids away from triglyceride synthesis and assimilation and toward fatty acid oxidation. Omega–3 lipids appear to have a unique ability to enhance thermogenesis and Essential Fatty Acids thereby reduce the efficiency of body fat deposition. EFAs exert their effects on lipid metabolism and thermogenesis by up-regulating the transcription of the mitochondrial uncoupling protein–3 (UCP3), and inducing genes encoding proteins involved in fatty acid oxidation (e.g. carnitine palmitoyltransferase and acyl–CoA oxidase) while simultaneously down-regulating the transcription of genes encoding proteins involved in lipid synthesis (e.g. fatty acid synthase).

A lack of EFAs—in particular the omega–3 EFAs—appears to be one of the dietary factors leading to the development of obesity and insulin resistance seen in Syndrome X (see section on Chromium for more information on Syndrome X).

Of particular interest, the body makes something called prostaglandins (as well as other highly unsaturated compounds) from both of the essential fatty acids. Prostaglandins are highly active, short-lived, hormone-like substances that regulate cellular activity on a moment-to-moment basis. Prostaglandins are directly involved with regulating blood pressure, inflammatory responses, insulin sensitivity, immune responses, anabolic/catabolic processes, and hundreds of other functions known and yet unknown.

The long and the short of all this, without going into a long and boring biochemical explanation: omega–3 fatty acids are responsible for forming the anti-inflammatory prostaglandins, and omega–6 derived prostaglandins are responsible for making many of the pro-inflammatory prostaglandins (in addition to other products derived from EFAs—of which there are many).

Obviously, it's a lot more complicated than that, but hey, I only have so much space to write…

What does the research say for athletic performance?

For the purposes of this book, where essential fatty acids are most useful is for optimizing body composition. Research has shown omega–3 fatty acids added to the diets of animals such as rats, mice, and pigs, results in fat loss. Many in vitro (test tube) studies also have been very clear as to the effects of flax oil (and other oils high in omega–3 fatty acids) on fat loss and other health related issues. There have been human studies that suggest flax oil can help with weight loss but there are no "smoking gun" type studies to convince the hardcore skeptic.

I wish I could show people the huge pile of research I have gathered over the years that demonstrate just how interesting and effective oils high in omega–3 fatty acids can be for weight loss, health, and overall well-being. Not all the research agrees (and it never does) but the vast majority of studies strongly suggest the omega–3 fatty acids from flax seed oil, fish oil, etc., are very effective for weight loss, with new studies coming out regularly. A few recent studies have found some mild performance effects with fish oil, but again, it's not something that should have a major impact there.

We need more human research to confirm this weight loss effect to the satisfaction of many scientists, but it's my opinion the data is more than satisfactory to recommend it.

Most of the research over the years has in fact been done on the fish oils, and many people are already aware of such research. Flax oil and other high ALA oils have been more recently studied. The human body can, in fact, make the DHA and EPA preformed in fish oil from the ALA found in flax oil (via desaturase enzymes), but some controversy still exists as to how efficiently it's converted which is why some still recommend fish oils over flax.

Some studies suggest the conversion of ALA (found in flax) to EPA and DHA (the "fish oils") is more efficient then commonly believed. One study called "Dietary substitution with an alpha–linolenic acid rich vegetable oil increases eicosapentaenoic acid (EPA) concentrations in tissues" examined this issue.

This study took thirty healthy volunteers and separated them into two groups. Group one ate a high ALA and low LA diet. The other group ate a high LA and low ALA diet, which is more typical of the average American's diet. The study ran for eight weeks, which is a relatively short time. At the end of four weeks the group receiving a high ALA and low LA diet had significantly higher levels of EPA in their plasma lipid fractions than the group receiving a high LA/low ALA diet.

For another four weeks both groups were given fish oil supplements. The group that got the flax oil and fish oil supplements had far higher levels of EPA than the group getting fish oil without the flax oil leading researchers to conclude:

" ...the results indicate that alpha–linolenic acid rich vegetable oils can be used in a domestic setting (in conjunction with a background diet low in LA) to elevate EPA in tissues to concentrations comparable with those associated with fish oil supplementation."

This is only one of several studies that found ingesting flax oil does raise EPA in tissues reliably and predictably. This does not mean preformed EPA and DHA don't have their uses, and one study that fed people 6 grams of fish oil per day found significant weight loss.

In my experience, flax oil is quite effective for fat loss and providing other health benefits. In my view, there may be reasons not to use the fish oils as the sole source of omega–3 fats. They are far more susceptible to oxidation and rancidity. The production of fish oils for use as a supplement is not as well controlled as for flax seed oil and fish oils can contain toxins such as PCBs and other compounds. Fish oils do have their therapeutic uses however.

What about real world athletic performance?

In the vast majority of people who have added flax oil to their diet (or other oils high in omega–3 fatty acids), improved fat loss has been the result. How much fat loss seems to be fairly individual and depends on many factors and physiological variables such as diet, exercise, initial fatty acid status, and body fat levels.

Fish oil supplements also get high marks for fat loss with most people as covered below.

Will Brink's Recommendation

Flax oil has been a particular interest of mine for years. As some people may already know, I was the first person to popularize the use of flax oil with bodybuilders and other athletes for fat loss.

As I hope you can appreciate, I have attempted to distill a great deal of complicated information regarding the essential fatty acids and their effects on fat loss in this section, and I have of course left out a considerable amount of information in order to get to the point and offer a simple recommendation, but, with what's here you should certainly get the gist of it.

I generally tell people to take 1-3 tablespoons of flax oil per day mixed in a protein drink, put over a salad with some vinegar, or taken straight from the bottle.

Don't bother with the capsules as it takes 12-14 capsules to equal one tablespoon, which becomes expensive and inconvenient.

Granted, I know most people don't like vague advice and request a specific figure. So, I recommend one tablespoon of flax oil for every 75 lb of body weight, though more can be used if desired. In fact, many "large and in charge" high level bodybuilders take up to seven tablespoons of flax oil a day before a contest and were still losing body fat on that much oil! People do not get fat on flax oil, period.

Ill informed nutritionists who tell you "all fats will make you fat and should be avoided" are simply incorrect and have not done their homework. There are a few points to consider regarding flax oil.

First of all, flax oil—like all polyunsaturated oils—is very sensitive to heat, light, and oxygen. It should never be heated or cooked with and should be kept in the fridge after opening the bottle.

Secondly, when a person increases their intake of such oils, they should also increase their intake of antioxidants such as vitamin C, E, selenium, and others. A good antioxidant complex is recommended.

Finally, there is a drawback to taking large amounts of flax for long periods of time, and that is the possibility that one could end up with a deficiency in the omega–6 EFAs.

What to do?

Several companies have developed oil products to address the issue of potential imbalances from long term flax oil intake. For example, Dr. Erasmus (the fat guru) has a product aptly named Udo's Choice™ Oil Blend. (Note: long before the bodybuilding community became aware of the importance of EFA's for fat loss—thanks in large part to yours truly—Dr. Erasmus was extolling the virtues of the essential fatty acids for health, fat loss, and performance.)

As previously mentioned flax oil is particularly rich in omega–3 essential fatty acids (ALA) but is actually a poor source of the omega–6 fatty acid, LA. This makes flax oil "omega–3 rich" and "omega–6 poor" for long term use. Many writers on nutrition have made the mistake of telling people that flax oil is a good source of the essential fatty acids, which is not true. It is a good source of the omega–3 essential fatty acids but lacks adequate omega–6 EFAs for long term use.

There are two schools of thought on how to look at this problem. One says that most people already eat far too much omega–6 oils (which they do) and far too little omega–3 oils (also correct), and taking flax oil will bring you into balance. The other believes flax oil is too rich in omega–3 essential fatty acids and taking it exclusively will lead to an omega–6 deficiency.

Where do I stand on this issue? I think both assumptions are correct depending on the population (or individual) you are looking at. What various companies have done is alter the ratio of omega–3 to omega–6 by mixing different oils together to get something closer to a 2:1 ratio of omega–3 to omega–6, as opposed to the 4:1 ratio of flax oil. What this does is bring the ratio closer to what is optimal (and avoids any imbalances) while keeping it an omega–3 rich product that we find gets the best results. In addition, several companies have added other important and useful ingredients for health and fatty acid metabolism such as: lecithin, vitamin E, GLA, etc.

As you can see from the above discussion, not only do we need to get adequate amounts of both the essential fatty acids (ALA and LA), but we need to take them in the proper ratios with respect to one another. I have recently seen some of the companies that make these types of products, producing oils in a 1:1 ratio of ALA to LA, but I definitely prefer a product with more emphasis on the omega–3 essential fatty acids. I have seen much better results in health, fat loss, and muscle gains, from an omega–3 rich product.

Perhaps the best way of getting maximum benefits from such products is to use them most of the time, throwing in a bottle of flax once in a while. The person can then switch over to flax oil exclusively during specific times when losing fat is the immediate goal.

I have found using this strategy with bodybuilders before contests is an optimal solution, and I consider this strategy the best of all possible worlds. I have gotten some pretty impressive results with it. A person can, of course, make their own oil blend with various ALA and LA ratios by mixing LA rich oils with the flax oil, but products such as Udo's Choice™ just makes life easier, and many such products contain other useful ingredients.

As far as bang for your buck, flax oil and other oil blends are about the best weight loss health/improving product around in my humble opinion. As for fish oils, my advice is to eat at least two to three servings per week of fish known to be high in healthy fish oils, such as salmon, tuna, and others.

There are now all manner of mixed oil products out there such as Udo's Choice™, and oils with different ratios of EFAs, such as Hemp, as well as others. There are also products such as Udo's + DHA, which uses an algal derived form of DHA, so it's close to a best of both worlds combination that would be excellent for vegetarians.

The inevitable comparison: fish oils vs. flax:

So you read the above, and have the inevitable question "do I take flax or fish oils?" If following diet to lose fat specifically, I recommend you use fish oils. The reason is not because on is qualitatively superior to the other per se, but because fish oil is a much more concentrated source of the "active" pre formed lipids EPA and DHA, which means far fewer fat calories coming from the fish oil, which gives you much more wiggle room with your fat calories when on low calorie intakes.

If using flax as the source of omega 3 lipids, you need considerably more of it to get the same amount of "active lipids" which makes is harder to fit other fats into your diet from the foods you eat and or from other sources, such as olive oil, etc. Thus, if following a diet to lose fat, which means you will be in a calorie deficit and need to be careful with your fat sources, I recommend using fish oils.

However, if not in a calories deficit, then using flax or Udo's or some other blended oil product is fine. Personally for example, I use both. I will cut my fish oil dose in half, and add Udo's or flax oil into my diet if not attempting to lose fat, which means my calorie intake is higher and I have more room to play with fat calories. So, when dieting, use fish oil, and get your other fats from naturally occurring sources from the foods you eat, small amounts of olive oil, etc and when not dieting/eating higher calories, use flax/Udo's or both (flax + fish, Udo's + fish, Hemp + fish, etc.), as it fits into your calorie requirements.

Flax, and other EFA rich oils, get an unqualified thumbs up from me, but must be used intelligently, depending on total calorie intakes and goals.

"But I still want to know more about fish oils!" you say? OK...

ф

FISH OIL

What is it?

As the name implies, oils derived from fish. That's the easy part to remember. The "active" omega–3 lipids found in fish oil are EPA eicosapentaenoic acid (EPA) and docosahexaenoic acid (DHA). EPA and DHA are the "active" fatty acids that come pre formed in fish, or can be can be converted in the human body from the essential fatty acid Linoleic acid (LA).

Before you raise your hand to ask exactly what is an essential fatty acid, where does this LA come from, and so on, that topic is fully covered in the section on flax oil, so don't concern yourself with it in this section. In this section, I examine "fish oils"—which contain the active lipids EPA/DHA—specifically, and will fill in additional questions the reader may have in the following section on flax oil.

What is it supposed to do?

The term "omega–3 fatty acid" should ring a bell for you. Fish oils are well publicized omega–3 fatty acids that have been shown to have many benefits.

While the list of potential health benefits of fish oils is extensive and beyond the scope of this section, I'll give you the short story; EPA and DHA are essential to brain and nervous system function development, may help treat and or reduce the risk of developing arthritis, high blood pressure, various cancers, and heart disease.

And that's just the tip of the iceberg! Omega–3 fatty acids are anti-lipogenic (they block fat storage), anti-catabolic, anti-inflammatory, they increase beta oxidation (fat burning!), improve insulin sensitivity, increase thermogenesis, and a whole lot more positive effects on health we don't have the space, time, or need, to cover in this section. However, as fat loss is our focus here, I will limit the discussion to that topic from here on.

Other studies find it may help with ADD, ADHD, depression, and autism! Yet other studies find fish oils may help relieve back and neck pain.

Interestingly, research has found the omega–3 lipids control gene transcription. (the more technically adept readers will have an interest in the below piece):

Omega–3 lipids play essential roles in the maintenance of energy balance and function as fuel partitioners in that they direct glucose toward glycogen storage, and direct fatty acids away from triglyceride synthesis and assimilation and toward fatty acid oxidation. Omega–3 lipids appear to have the unique ability to enhance thermogenesis and thereby reduce the efficiency of body fat deposition. EFAs exert their effects on lipid metabolism and thermogenesis by upregulating the transcription of the mitochondrial uncoupling protein–3, and inducing genes encoding proteins involved in fatty acid oxidation (e.g. carnitine palmitoyltransferase and acyl–CoA oxidase) while simultaneously down-regulating the transcription of genes encoding proteins involved in lipid synthesis (e.g. fatty acid synthase).

A lack of omega–3 lipids appears to be one of the dietary factors leading to the development of obesity and insulin resistance seen in Syndrome X (see section on Chromium for more information of Syndrome X). Finally, studies also find fish oil raises resting energy expenditure (REE) which should improve fat loss over time.

What does the research have to say?

Research has shown omega–3 fatty acids added to the diets of animals such as rats, mice, and pigs, results in fat loss. In animal studies, the effect has been quite consistent. However, studies in humans with fish oils have suggested only moderate effects on fat loss or have been inconsistent.

One study presented at the North American Association for Study of Obesity (NAASO) Annual Meeting gave 20 obese women (Body Mass Index above 40) fish oil supplements. The women were already on a very low calorie diet, with one group getting fish oil and another getting placebo. The group given the omega–3 supplements had a 20% greater weight loss than the group given placebo after only three weeks with BMI reduced by as much as 15%. That's one of the more impressive studies done with fish oils in people, and it may be an effect seen in a specific population of obese women severely lacking any omega–3 fats in their diets, but still interesting.

It should be noted however that not all studies in humans have been so dramatic, and that may be due to doses used, nutritional status of the study group, activity levels, and other variables. For example, another study with 6 men replaced 6 grams per day of dietary fats from other sources following a control diet. They had 6 grams of fat replaces in their diet with 6 g of fish oil which was equal to 1.1 gram of DHA and 0.7 grams of EPA, for a total of 1.8 g of "active" lipids from fish oil. These men were allowed to eat their normal diets as they wished (ad libitum) for 12 weeks taking the fish oil supplements 3 times per day.

Their body weights did not change. However, their body composition did change slightly, with a 2 lb loss of fat and an impressive 25% increase in beta oxidation (fat burning!) which over time, may have resulted in additional fat loss. A few lbs of fat loss (which didn't reach statistical significance) is not terribly impressive granted, but when you factor in the fact they were not on a diet or exercising, as well the big increase in fat oxidation rates, it's a worthwhile study to note.

The research has been generally favorable with fish oils in humans, though not as dramatic as the first study mentioned above.

What does the real world have to say?

In the vast majority of people who have added fish oils to their diet, improved fat loss has been the result. How much fat loss seems to be fairly individual and depends on many factors and physiological variables such as diet, exercise, initial fatty acid status, dose, and body fat levels. Fish oils are one of those supplements where the real world effects seem to consistently outpace what the research finds, as least where fat loss is concerned. Feedback for fish oils is almost universally positive.

Recommendations

In the past I had reservations about recommending fish oils. I wrote:

"In my view, there are reasons not to use the fish oils as the sole source of omega–3 fats. They are far more susceptible to oxidation and rancidity. The production of fish oils for use as a supplement is not as well controlled as for flax seed oil and fish oils can contain toxins such as PCBs and other compounds. Fish oils do have their therapeutic uses."

The quality of fish oil supplements across the spectrum of products has improved greatly in the past few years with the use of processing techniques such molecular distillation and others, which produces very high quality fish oil products. Of the major brands, such as The Life Extension® Foundation, Nordic Naturals®, and Carlson®, I would not worry much about that issue any more. I no longer have the above concerns for fish oil supplements, which is a good thing, considering how useful and healthy these products are.

On the issue of doses, recall, it's not the amount of fish oil you take in, it's the amount if "active" lipids in the fish oil; EPA and DHA.

Obviously, 6 caps of fish oil containing 40% total active lipids is going to be a different dose than 6 caps containing 30% active lipids, so you must read the labels for EPA and DHA content per cap. In general, 30% active lipids—the combined amount of EPA and DHA in the product—is typical of most brands, but fish oil products with a higher percentage do exist, they just cost more but allow you to take fewer caps.

How much should you take?

Studies have used doses that are quite variable, so no exact dose is known in terms of optimal effects on fat loss, but 6 - 10 g/day (assuming 30% EPA + DHA) is a starting point. So, a 1000 mg (1 g) softgell cap of fish oil, would be approximately 180 mg of EPA and 120 mg of DHA, assuming the general rule of 30% total active lipids. Fish oil comes as 60/40 EPA to DHA.

I would recommend at least approximately 6 g (6 1000 mg caps) fish oils giving you a total of 1800 mg of active lipids per day assuming 30% of 6 g is EPA and DHA, but you must read the labels for exact numbers.

Looking at specific brands for example:

Puritan's Pride®: They use a 1200 mg cap, each containing 360 mg total active lipids. You would need 5 caps to equal 1800 mg total active lipids.

The Life Extension® Foundation: They use a 1000 mg cap that gives 600 mg total active lipids per cap, which means you would need 3 caps to equal the recommended 1800 mg above.

Nordic Naturals®: they use a 1000 mg cap that gives a total of 275 mg of active lipids per cap, so you will need 6-7 caps per day

Carlson®: they use a 1000 mg cap that gives a total of 320 mg of active Omega–3 lipids, so you would need 5-6 caps of this product.

Liquid versus gelcaps

Several companies make liquid versions of their fish oil products, which can be both convenient and cost effective. There's no reason not to use the liquid versions if you don't mind the taste and you remember to read the labels for total active omega–3 lipid content. For example, Carlson® makes a lemon favored liquid product that contains approximately the required amount of EPA and DHA in one teaspoon, so that's convenient and cost effective.

Higher doses versus regular dose

Can one use higher doses than listed above? Absolutely, and many do. Are higher doses more effective for fat loss? Unclear, but many feel higher doses are more effective, although the data is lacking there. If one uses higher doses, you will have to adjust calorie and fat intakes to account for much higher doses. At the amount recommended in this section, the added calories are negligible, but at 10,000 mg (10 g) and higher, the additional fat and calorie content will need to be accounted for. That's not a negative per se, just something that does add additional complexity to your calorie and fat calculations during a fat loss phase.

Finally, although I'm sure I don't really need to say this at this point, fish oils get a thumbs up from me and I consider them an essential product during a diet.

References

Mason CM, Long J, Conroy C. Prescription Omega–3s: An Overview for Nurse Practitioners. The Journal of cardiovascular nursing 2011;26(4):290-97.

Carpentier YA, Portois L, Malaisse WJ. n–3 fatty acids and the metabolic syndrome. Am J Clin Nutr. 2006 Jun;83(6 Suppl):1499S-1504S.

Flachs P, Horakova O, Brauner P, et al. Polyunsaturated fatty acids of marine origin upregulate mitochondrial biogenesis and induce beta–oxidation in white fat. Diabetologia. 2005 Nov;48(11):2365-75.

Ide T. Effect of dietary alpha–linolenic acid on the activity and gene expression of hepatic fatty acid oxidation enzymes. Biofactors. 2000;13(1-4):9-14.

Ide T, Kobayashi H, Ashakumary L, et al. Comparative effects of perilla and fish oils on the activity and gene expression of fatty acid oxidation enzymes in rat liver. Biochim Biophys Acta. 2000 May 6;1485(1):23-35.

Lombardo YB, Chicco AG. Effects of dietary polyunsaturated n–3 fatty acids on dyslipidemia and insulin resistance in rodents and humans. A review. J Nutr Biochem. 2006 Jan;17(1):1-13.

Mantzioris E, James MJ, Gibson RA, Cleland LG. Dietary substitution with an alpha–linolenic acid–rich vegetable oil increases eicosapentaenoic acid concentrations in tissues. Am J Clin Nutr. 1994 Jun;59(6):1304-9.

Oudart H, Groscolas R, Calgari C, et al. Brown fat thermogenesis in rats fed high–fat diets enriched with n–3 polyunsaturated fatty acids. International Journal of Obesity and Related Metabolic Disorders. 1997 Nov;21(11):955-62.

Rossi AS, Lombardo YB, Lacorte JM, et al. Dietary fish oil positively regulates plasma leptin and adiponectin levels in sucrose–fed, insulin–resistant rats. Am J Physiol Regul Integr Comp Physiol. 2005 Aug;289(2):R486-R494.

Ruzickova J, Rossmeisl M, Prazak T, et al. Omega–3 PUFA of marine origin limit diet–induced obesity in mice by reducing cellularity of adipose tissue.Lipids. 2004 Dec;39(12):1177-85.

♉

VANADYL SULPHATE

What is it?

Vanadium is a trace mineral found in small quantities in various foods with seafood, mushrooms, various cereals and soybeans, being the richest sources of this mineral. Vanadyl sulphate (often spelled sulfate) is the sulfur-bound form of the mineral. Vanadium can also be bound to other compounds, but the sulphate (a vanadium salt) is the one most often seen in supplement form.

What is it supposed to do?

Vanadium is similar to chromium (see chromium section) in its effects and mechanisms of action, Vanadium plays a direct role in the metabolism of carbohydrates and the regulation of blood sugar, as well as having effects on cholesterol and blood lipid metabolism. Vanadium is often referred to as an 'insulin mimicker' as it appears to be able to mimic the actions of insulin on various tissues. In athletes, the interest in vanadyl sulphate is related to its insulin mimicking mechanisms, such as possible effects on glycogen synthesis and muscle anabolism. In diabetics, vanadium supplements may have a positive effect in regulating blood glucose levels, as well as having effects on glycosylated hemoglobin levels in people with non–insulin dependent diabetes mellitus (NIDDM).

In bodybuilders and other strength training athletes it's claimed vanadyl sulphate makes muscles fuller due (one assumes) to the possible increased glycogen storage.

What does the research say for athletic performance?

The research with vanadium compounds has, as one might expect, focused mostly on its effects on diabetes. In both diabetics humans and animals, vanadium generally has positive effects on blood sugar regulation, hepatic insulin resistance, and other outcomes important to diabetics. Studies looking at the effects in healthy people are less dramatic. Few studies exist that look specifically at vanadium in healthy people and its effects on strength or body composition in particular.

What does exist is not impressive. A study done in 1996 called "The effect of oral vanadyl sulfate on body composition and performance in weight-training athletes" found no significant effects on strength or bodycomposition. This was a 12 week, double-blind, placebo-controlled trial involving weight training volunteers. The researchers looked at both 1 rep max and 10 rep max, as well as any body composition changes between the group getting the vanadyl sulphate and the placebo group. Thirty one subjects completed the 12 week trial, so it was a decent sized study that ran long enough to provide valuable information. It was concluded that:

" ...oral vanadyl sulfate was ineffective in changing body composition in weight–training athletes, and any modest performance–enhancing effect requires further investigation"

What does the real world say?

Vanadyl sulphate had a short run as a popular supplement over a decade ago. It went the way of the Dodo bird in popularity due to the fact it didn't seem to work as claimed. Some people have reported they thought their muscles felt fuller, but that's about the most positive feedback I have gotten over the years.

Will Brink's Recommendation

When vanadyl sulphate first came out, there were some serious safety concerns. But, studies don't seem to find acute toxicity with this supplement at doses normally used by people to improve glucose metabolism. At doses of 100 mg per day, gastrointestinal side effects are common. It should be noted that all of the trace minerals, such as iron, chromium, and zinc, become toxic at high enough doses. The typical dose found in sports nutrition products provide 20-50 mg per day of vanadyl sulphate.

For people with diabetes, vanadyl sulphate may be of some use in blood sugar regulation and potentially reducing the need for insulin. If you have diabetes, make sure to consult your doctor before using this supplement.

In healthy athletes looking to add strength or LBM, vanadyl sulphate gets a big thumbs down from me. Money is far better spent on other supplements covered in this book.

References

Boden G et al. Effects of vanadyl sulfate on carbohydrate and lipid metabolism in patients with non–insulin–dependent diabetes mellitus. Metabolism. 1996 Sep;45(9):1130-5.

Cam MC, et al. Long–term effectiveness of oral vanadyl sulphate in streptozotocin–diabetic rats. Diabetologia. 1993 Mar;36(3):218-24.

Fawcett JP, et al. The effect of oral vanadyl sulfate on body composition and performance in weight–training athletes. Int J Sport Nutr. 1996 Dec;6(4):382-90.

Goldfine AB, Patti ME, Zuberi L, et al. Metabolic effects of vanadyl sulfate in humans with non–insulin–dependent diabetes mellitus: in vivo and in vitro studies. Metabolism. 2000 Mar;49(3):400-10.

Jentjens RL, Jeukendrup AE. Effect of acute and short–term administration of vanadyl sulphate on insulin sensitivity in healthy active humans. Int J Sport Nutr Exerc Metab. 2002 Dec;12(4):470-9.

Shafrir E, et al. Treatment of diabetes with vanadium salts: general overview and amelioration of nutritionally induced diabetes in the Psammomys obesus gerbil. Diabetes Metab Res Rev. 2001 Jan–Feb;17(1):55-66.

Srivastava AK. Anti–diabetic and toxic effects of vanadium compounds. Mol Cell Biochem. 2000 Mar;206(1-2):177-82.

Tsunajima T, Tatsuki R, Satoh K, et.al. Improvement of impaired glucose tolerance by oral administration of vanadyl sulfate by gavage in streptozotocin–induced diabetic rats. Res Commun Mol Pathol Pharmacol. 1997 Nov;98(2):190-200.

ℊ

VITAMIN C

What is it?

Vitamin C is an essential nutrient for only a few animals, including humans. Vitamin C can be synthesized from glucose in most plants and animals, but humans (and other vitamin C requiring animals) lack L–gulono–gamma–lactone oxidase, the enzyme catalyzing the final step in the biosynthetic pathway.

What is it supposed to do?

Most people know vitamin C (ascorbic acid) as a simple vitamin and antioxidant needed for optimal health. They would be right. Vitamin C is a water-soluble antioxidant in the human body and plays a wide variety of roles in metabolism, ranging from immunity to hormone production.

What does the research say for athletic performance?

Vitamin C may also play additional roles above and beyond its simple role as an essential nutrient found in our diet and supplements.

Although exercise has been shown to improve antioxidant mechanisms, one well known side effect is that it raises oxidative stress and increases free radical production. Defenses can be overwhelmed over time and the risks of increased free radical production are well known, such as damage to DNA and a host of pathologies best avoided. When we factor in our various life styles and the environment, the issue of free radical production and oxidative stress is made more important.

Some studies have reported that supplementation with vitamins C and E, or antioxidant mixtures, can reduce oxidative stress from intense exercise and trained athletes who received antioxidant supplements show evidence of reduced oxidative stress.

Like all things in life, there is always a flip side and exercise is no exception. Though the benefits clearly outweigh the risks, we must acknowledge the potential downsides, or problems associated with exercise, and look for ways to minimize them. Although moderate exercise has been shown to improve immunity, extreme and prolonged exercise has been shown to suppress the immune system.

This is commonly called, "over training syndrome" or OTS, and is common with athletes who train too long, too hard and too often. OTS is also found in elite military groups such as the US Navy Seals who are forced to train under extreme conditions.

One study found that a group of runners who trained for a marathon, but did not compete, was much less likely to get upper respiratory infections than the runners who completed the race, showing how much such endeavors can take out of a person.

Vitamin C has been shown to reduce oxidative stress and suppress levels of the muscle wasting hormone cortisol, as well as prevent the decline in immunity after intense exercise, but, all studies do not agree on these effects of vitamin C, or on antioxidants in general, on immunity.

Athletes should not view taking additional vitamin C as a direct performance enhancer per se, but as a long term preventative nutrient essential to long term health. Without good health, clearly, performance will suffer.

So, indirectly, adequate vitamin C intakes are important for long term performance, although studies don't find positive effects on short term performance.

What about real world athletic performance?

Anecdotally, there are some who feel taking higher doses of vitamin C have been helpful for boosting immunity to colds and other upper respiratory infections.

Will Brink's Recommendation

Exactly what the "optimal" intake of vitamin C remains to be elucidated, but there appears to be no health risks associate with taking higher amounts than the RDA recommend. Individual intakes of vitamin C can range dramatically, from 100 mg per day to several thousand milligrams, with most studies looking at "high dose C" using between 200 and 1000 mg per day.

Although there is not an optimal dose known at this time, 200-500 mg daily of vitamin C added to an athletes diet is a common dose and should be adequate. For general health and well-being, vitamin C gets a big thumbs up, but for direct effects on building muscle or improving performance, it has to get a thumbs down.

References

Schroder H, Navarro E et al. Nutrition antioxidant status and oxidative stress in professional basketball players: effects of a three compound antioxidative supplement. Int J Sports Med. 2000 Feb;21(2):146-50.

Balakrishnan SD, Anuradha CV. Exercise, depletion of antioxidants and antioxidant manipulation. Cell Biochem Funct. 1998 Dec;16(4):269-75.

Peters EM. Exercise, immunology and upper respiratory tract infections. Int J Sports Med. 1997 Mar;18 Suppl 1:S69-77.

φ

VITAMIN E

What is it?

Vitamin E actually refers to a family of structurally related compounds: alpha, beta, delta and gamma tocopherols, and alpha, beta, delta, and gamma tocotrienols. All are biologically active, although alpha–tocopherol is the form maintained in plasma, and is the one most likely to be found in multivitamins and other supplements and fortified foods. Most of the research studies to date on the benefits of vitamin E have focused on the alpha–tocopherol form, which is the only one for which an RDA has been established.

What is it supposed to do?

Vitamin E supplements are taken to mitigate oxidative stress.

What does the research say for athletic performance?

Most of what was said about vitamin C will be similar for vitamin E. As with C, people are familiar with vitamin E as a simple vitamin and antioxidant needed for optimal health.

Vitamin E is the major fat soluble antioxidant in the human body and plays a wide variety of roles in metabolism, ranging from immunity to fertility to hormone production. As with all antioxidants, vitamin E works in conjunction with other antioxidants such as vitamin C, glutathione, selenium, and beta–carotenes, as well as with key antioxidant enzymes, such as superoxide dismutase, glutathione peroxidase, and catalase.

As mentioned in the vitamin C section—although exercise has been shown to improve antioxidant mechanisms, one well known side effect is that it raises oxidative stress and increases free radical production. Defenses can be overwhelmed over time and the risks of increased free radical production is well known, such as damage to DNA, reduced immunity, susceptibility to upper respiratory infections and other potential health problems best avoided. When we factor in our various life styles and environment (e.g., pollution, ozone, etc) the issue of free radical production and oxidative stress is made more important.

Some studies have reported that supplementation with vitamin E and/or antioxidant mixtures, can reduce oxidative stress from intense exercise and trained athletes who received antioxidant supplements show evidence of reduced oxidative stress. Studies with vitamin E that have looked directly at athletic performance have been contradictory, with most studies finding no direct effects on performance.

Vitamin E has been shown to reduce oxidative stress. In particular, because vitamin E is fat soluble, it helps to prevent something called exercise induced lipid peroxidation.

For example, one recent study evaluated the effects of 5 months of vitamin E (alpha–tocopherol) supplementation on physical performance during aerobic exercise training in 30 top class cyclists. The study found the plasma vitamin E concentration increased significantly in the vitamin E supplemented group, whereas the placebo group showed a trend toward decrease.

The study also found statistically significant drops in biochemical indices of oxidative stress in the group getting the vitamin E. But they did not find direct improvements in performance in the vitamin E group over that of placebo.

Some studies suggest vitamin E can prevent the decline in immunity after intense exercise. but it should be noted that not all studies agree on these effects of vitamin E or antioxidants, in general, on immunity.

It is interesting to note that other members of the vitamin E family may also exert protective effects that are distinct from alpha–tocopherol. For example, gamma–tocopherol—unlike the alpha form—is able to scavenge nitrogen radicals which also can damage cells and tissues. More research is required to assess whether supplementing with other members of the vitamin E family confer more benefits than supplementing with alpha–tocopherol alone.

What about real world athletic performance?

No one I've spoken to has ever reported any direct gains or improved performance as a result of taking vitamin E.

Will Brink's Recommendation

Athletes should not view taking additional vitamin E as a direct performance enhancer per se, but as a long–term preventative nutrient, essential to long term health.

Good health is, after all, a prerequisite for performance over the long run. Clearly, adequate vitamin E intakes are important for long term performance, although studies don't find positive effects on short term performance.

What exactly is the optimal intake of vitamin E is unclear at this time, but there appears to be no health risks associate with taking higher amounts than the RDA—within reason.

Individual intakes of vitamin E vary dramatically, with most studies using between 200 IU to 800 IU per day. Although there is not an optimal dose known at this time, 400 IU to 800 IU appears safe and effective. The US Institute of Medicine has established a tolerable upper intake level (UL) for alpha–tocopherol of 1,500 IU/day for adults.

Even less is known about optimal intakes of gamma and other tocopherols, although some researchers have suggested that both the gamma and alpha forms should be used when conducting trials on the efficacy of vitamin E supplementation for cancer prevention.

For general health and well-being, vitamin E gets a thumbs up, but for any anabolic or performance enhancing effects, it gets a thumbs down.

References

Balakrishnan SD, Anuradha CV. Exercise, depletion of antioxidants and antioxidant manipulation. Cell Biochem Funct. 1998 Dec;16(4):269-75.

Helzlsouer KJ, Huang HY, Alberg AJ, Hoffman S, et al. Association between alpha–tocopherol, gamma–tocopherol, selenium, and subsequent prostate cancer. J Natl Cancer Inst. 2000 Dec 20;92(24):2018-23.

Powers SK, Hamilton K. Antioxidants and exercise. Clin Sports Med. 1999 Jul;18(3):525-36.

Rokitzki L, Logemann E, Huber G, Keck E, Keul J. Alpha–Tocopherol supplementation in racing cyclists during extreme endurance training. Int J Sport Nutr. 1994 Sep;4(3):253-64.

☧

ZMA

What is it?

ZMA is a supplement consisting of two amino acid-chelated minerals, zinc and magnesium, plus vitamin B6.

What is it supposed to do?

ZMA is claimed to raise the anabolic hormones testosterone and IGF–1, and possibly to improve performance in athletes.

What does the research say for athletic performance?

The claims are lofty, but are they true? The claims of such products rest on four basic premises:

1. Athletes are notoriously lacking in zinc and magnesium due to several factors, ranging from poor diets to increased usage/excretion of these minerals.

2. Zinc and magnesium are particularly important minerals in the production of anabolic (muscle building) hormones needed by athletes.

3. Due to competition during digestion, even the inclusion of a multivitamin and other mixed mineral supplements will not correct the deficiency.

4. These products are based on a particular form of zinc and magnesium (zinc monomethionine–aspartate and magnesium aspartate) which are superior to inorganic forms of the minerals. This brings us to ZMA.

That's the basic contention of this zinc and magnesium based product in a nut shell, with some biochemical twists and turns I am leaving out due to space limitations and to preserve the brain cells of you, the reader!

Looking at premise number one, there is a decent body of research that has indeed shown that zinc and magnesium deficiencies are not uncommon in various athletes, such as football players, cyclists, bodybuilders, and elite military groups.

Looking at premise number two, it is well established that these two minerals are needed in over 300 different enzymatic reactions and the production of testosterone is one of them.

Examining premise number three, there are several studies that examined the issue of nutrient interactions and, indeed, found that certain minerals compete for absorption and so, may not get absorbed if taken together. Several studies have found that even the addition of a multivitamin to the diet of people did not increase the levels of zinc, magnesium and other minerals, while the serum vitamin levels did go up. The authors theorized this was due to competition of the minerals in the multivitamin. So, it would appear that different minerals need to be taken at different times and taking them altogether may not be an optimal, or even effective, strategy for increasing levels of these minerals in tissues.

The fourth contention regarding the forms of minerals is a bit more unproven.

It's well known, that there is a wide range of absorption between different forms of nutrients, especially minerals, so the concept is not far fetched. The idea behind these supplements is to supply highly absorbable forms of non-competing minerals (in this case zinc and magnesium) known to be essential for the optimal production of anabolic hormones. Though a variety of companies are now selling this product, the letters ZMA appear in the name or on the bottle only if the product is using the patented ingredients.

We note the research done by a Dr. Brilla at Western Washington University. Dr. Brilla found the addition of 30 mg of zinc monomethionine–aspartate and 450 mg of magnesium aspartate (the forms used in ZMA) daily to football players had a 32 percent increase in total testosterone, a 3.6 percent increase in IGF–1, and improvements in strength levels.

However, more recent studies did not find ZMA to have any beneficial effects. Researchers of one study concluded

"...no significant differences were observed between groups in anabolic or catabolic hormone status, body composition, 1-RM bench press and leg press, upper or lower body muscular endurance, or cycling anaerobic capacity. Results indicate that ZMA supplementation during training does not appear to enhance training adaptations in resistance trained populations."

Another study published in the European Journal of Clinical Nutrition found that supplementation with ZMA did not have impact total or free testosterone.

What about real world athletic performance?

Some have reported modest gains in strength and performance with ZMA, although perhaps for an additional reason: ZMA is taken at bedtime, on an empty stomach. Taken this way, many insist that it helps them get a good night's sleep, and that reason alone is enough for many people to continue taking it.

Will Brink's Recommendation

With regard to the relationship between essential minerals and testosterone, one important caveat to remember with ZMA (or similar product) is that it will only work if there is a deficiency to correct. Supplementation will not increase levels of anabolic hormones where no deficiency in these minerals exists.

However, in light of more recent studies that do not appear to confirm earlier studies mentioned above, my early interest in this product is greatly tampered, and it must get a thumbs down at this time.

References

Koehler K, Parr MK, Geyer H, Mester J, Schänzer W. Serum testosterone and urinary excretion of steroid hormone metabolites after administration of a high-dose zinc supplement. Eur J Clin Nutr. 2009 Jan;63(1):65-70. Epub 2007 Sep 19.

Wilborn CD, et al. Effects of Zinc Magnesium Aspartate (ZMA) Supplementation on Training Adaptations and Markers of Anabolism and Catabolism. J Int Soc Sports Nutr. 2004 Dec 31;1(2):12-20

Brilla LR and Conte V. Novel Zinc and Magnesium Formulation (ZMA) Increases Anabolic Hormones and Strength in Athletes. JEPonline. 2000 Oct;3(4):26-36.

Prasad AS, Mantzoros CS, Beck FW, Hess JW, Brewer GJ. Zinc status and serum testosterone levels of healthy adults. Nutrition. 1996 May;12(5):344-8.

Singh A, Day BA, DeBolt JE, et al. Magnesium, Zinc and Copper status of US Navy SEAL Trainees. Am J Clin Nutr. 1989 Apr;49(4):695-700.

Telford RD, Catchpole EA, Deakin V, et al. The effect of 7 to 8 months of vitamin/mineral supplementation on the vitamin and mineral status of athletes. Int J Sport Nutr. 1992 Jun;2(2):123-34.

ቝ

Chapter

5

ANTI-ESTROGENS

The potentially negative effect of the "female" hormone estrogen is a constant concern for male athletes. Increased estrogen may lead to increases in body fat and other maladies athletes want to avoid (gyno, etc.) and many supplement companies have attempted to capitalize on this concern over excessive estrogen levels.

Anti-Estrogens Covered
❖ ATD
❖ Chrysin
❖ I3C/DIM
❖ 6–OXO

For example, some research suggests that supplements such as androstenedione, and a few of the other "andros," may increase estrogen levels by converting to estradiol (a powerful estrogen). Androgens such as testosterone and androstenedione convert to estradiol via an enzyme called "aromatase." Drugs or natural compounds that can block this enzyme are therefore called "anti-aromatase" agents.

Basically, there are two ways to affect estrogen. You can block the receptor site, or you can inhibit the enzyme (i.e. aromatase) that converts "male" hormones into "female" hormones (i.e. estrogens).

When a molecule fits into the receptor but does not send an estrogenic signal, it is called an "antagonist" meaning it prevents or "blocks" estrogen from getting to the receptor, but does not, in itself, act as an estrogen. Hence the term "estrogen blocker."

When something can lock into the receptor and does act as an estrogen, that is, activates the receptor to one degree or another, it's called an "agonist." So, an antagonist fits into a receptor (thus blocking something else from occupying that receptor) but does not activate the receptor and an agonist fits into the receptor in question (in this case an estrogen receptor) and does activate the receptor to one degree or another.

This is exactly how the drug Tamoxifen works when treating breast cancer. It can fit into the estrogen receptor, but does not activate it thus preventing estrogenic effects in the tissue in question.

Thus, Tamoxifen is an "estrogen antagonist." In truth, it's a bit more complicated than that as Tamoxifen is—in fact—both an estrogen antagonist or agonist depending in the tissue in question, which means it has mixed antagonist/agonist effects, but never mind...

So, what the reader should take away from the above is, you can block the effects of estrogen by either blocking the receptor it fits into, or inhibit the enzyme the body uses to convert androgens into estrogens. Got all that?

The use of anti-estrogen drugs and supplements is a part of post cycle therapy (PCT). PCT is a standard part of any anabolic steroid or prohormone cycle. PCT facilitates the transition to natural testosterone production following suppression by exogenous hormones.

Many people are more interested in simply boosting their own natural T production, and anti-estrogen supplements offer a means to do this. Some drug studies have demonstrated that—in principle—the concept is reasonably sound, although there is no information on the possible long term effects of doing this.

ATD

What is it?

3,17–dioxo–etiochol–1,4,6–triene (ATD) is an anti-aromatase with similar properties to 6–OXO in that is blocks the conversion of some androgens to estrogen via binding the aromatase enzyme. ATD also appears to have other effects beyond that of just its anti-estrogenic effects, such as (possible) selective anti-androgenic effects.

What is it supposed to do?

The claims for ATD are varied, but its major claim to fame is as an anti-estrogen that can increase testosterone levels. The mechanism by which ATD may increase testosterone is similar to that of 6–OXO (see 6–OXO section for further details and discussion on how anti-estrogens effect testosterone levels), so I will use what I wrote in the 6–OXO section to explain ATD's possible effects on testosterone and how it may achieve the effect…

"…by altering a key feedback loop in how the body regulates testosterone production."

Exactly how the body regulates various hormones is a very complex topic beyond the scope of this section. Suffice it to say, it primarily involves what's called the hypothalamic-pituitary-testicular axis (HPTA) which works via overlapping negative feedbackloops.

Estradiol is key in this system. Estradiol is suppressive to testosterone production. High estradiol sends the signal there is high testosterone, and T production is reduced. Lower estrogen, and the body thinks T is low, and sends the signal to produce more T. Reducing estrogen levels is a way to fool the HPTA into producing more T, via an increase in the gonadotropins: follicle stimulating hormone (FSH) and luteinizing hormone (LH) That's the basic mechanism, which has been greatly over simplified.

Articles and ads for this product claim ATD is "3 times more powerful than current popular anti-estrogen supplements" meaning it has 3 times the binding affinity over products such as 6–OXO.

Another mechanism by which ATD is claimed to increase testosterone is by binding to androgen receptors and acting as a possible Selective Androgen Receptor Modulator (S.A.R.M.).

The HPTA also responds to androgen levels as another part of the feedback loop. The H in the HPTA is key in this androgenic feedback mechanism. By binding to androgen receptors in the Hypothalamus (acting as a S.A.R.M) it's theorized that will fool the HPTA into thinking the body is low in androgens and increases the production of T.

That's the basic concept anyway.

What does the research say for athletic performance?

As you might expect, solid human data with ATD showing the aforementioned claimed effects is lacking. What exists is mostly older animal and in vitro (test tube) data, with some poorly controlled "in house" anecdotal information put out by the people/companies marketing ATD for controlling estrogen and or increasing T.

In animal and in vitro studies, ATD appears to be a compound with strong anti-aromatase properties. As mentioned, published in vivo human studies are lacking. It's supposed effects as a S.A.R.M are more interesting and even less proven in humans.

This is where things are going to get a tad complicated, but a needed background conversation is required to discuss the supposed S.A.R.M activity of ATD.

So what is a S.A.R.M and how does that apply to you? For this background conversation to happen, I am going to borrow information I wrote for the Saw Palmetto section regarding concepts such as receptor agonists, antagonists, mixed receptor activities, etc. in hopes of bringing it all together to explain what a S.A.R.M is, and whether or not ATD is even a S.A.R.M!

Some studies suggest ATD is simply an anti-androgen. That is, it binds to the androgen receptor (AR) on tissues but does not itself act as an androgen, which means it's acting as an AR antagonist or "AR blocker."

When a molecule (in this case ATD) fits into the AR but does not send a signal it is called an "antagonist," meaning it prevents or "blocks" a hormone (in this case testosterone) from getting to the receptor but does not in itself act as androgen as testosterone would normally. Hence the term "anti-androgen." When something can lock into the receptor and does act on the AR, that is activates the receptor to one degree or another, it's called an "agonist." So, an antagonist fits into a receptor (thus blocking something else from occupying that receptor) but does not activate the receptor and an agonist fits into the receptor in question and does activate the receptor to one degree or another.

Got all that?

Ah, but that's still not the entire story to explain what a S.A.R.M is. For example, let's take the drug Tamoxifen (brand name Nolvadex) as an example, which is not a S.A.R.M, but a SERM, or Selective Estrogen Receptor Modulator. It can fit into the estrogen receptor but does not activate it thus preventing estrogenic effects in the tissue in question. Drugs like Nolvadex, which have "mixed" antagonist and agonist properties are referred to as a SERM.

Just because something has anti-estrogenic effects on one tissue does not mean it will have that effect on all tissues.

A S.A.R.M would have the same mixed effects; it may act as an anti-androgen in one tissue while acting as a pro–androgen (or agonist) in other tissues. Research looking at legitimate S.A.R.Ms is a big area of research right now with several S.A.R.M drugs not far from being released to the market. A true S.A.R.M might have anti-androgenic effects on prostate tissue but act as an agonist on muscle tissue, which means the user might experience increased muscle mass without the side effects (such as potential increased risk of prostate enlargement) associated with androgens such as anabolic steroids and high doses of testosterone.

Where does that leave us with ATD? Most studies suggest ATD acts as androgen receptor antagonist (i.e. as an anti-androgen blocking the receptor that testosterone binds to at the surface of the cell) and this would not be what an athlete wants trying to gain muscle.

But, some studies also suggest it may act like a S.A.R.M. The theory put forth by companies selling ATD is that ATD acts differently at the level of the hypothalamus than it does on muscle tissue.

For example, one author claims that

"ATD has 90% androgenic activity in muscle and 10% in hypothalamus"

thus according to this author

"ATD tricks your hypothalamus into thinking your testosterone levels are low"

which will lead to an increase in testosterone production. My research of the literature does not substantiate these numbers and I could find no support for those specific figures or claims.

What about real world athletic performance?

As ATD is relatively new to the OTC market, I have gotten no real feedback on it.

Will Brink's Recommendation

As the reader can plainly see, the issue of ATD is a complex one with more unknowns than known effects in humans. Like 6–OXO,

ATD may have uses for estrogen control or as post cycle therapy after using AAS or prohormones, (which are no longer legal anyway….) etc. But at the moment, it's simply unclear what effects ATD has on testosterone levels, estrogen levels, and other effects in humans to recommend it at this time.

For example, if the net effect of ATD is as an anti-androgen in humans, it would not be what athletes want. If the theory that it acts as a S.A.R.M is true, it could very well benefit those who want increase testosterone levels. Bottom line is it's simply unclear what is going on with ATD and I recommend people avoid it until far more is known. It gets a thumbs down from me at this time.

Finally, the issue is now moot as this supplement is no longer legal to sell in the US, although there are batches of it floating around I hear (which is why I left this section in the book) and I recommend people avoid any gray market brands of this supplement.

References

Kaplan ME, McGinnis MY. Effects of ATD on male sexual behavior and androgen receptor binding: a reexamination of the aromatization hypothesis. Horm Behav. 1989 Mar;23(1):10-26.

ᚠ

CHRYSIN

What is it?

Chrysin is 5,7–dihydroxyflavone, a flavonoid found in large concentrations in Passiflora (Passionflower). Flavonoids are naturally occurring compounds found in plants that possess a variety of biological activities, including antioxidant activity.

What is it supposed to do?

Chrysin has been marketed as an anti-aromatase, or enzyme inhibitor. Chrysin is sold alone, or often added to other supplements, in hopes it will prevent any estrogen production that may result from taking prohormone or other hormone based supplements. Chrysin is a bioflavonoid similar to other flavonoids such as quercetin.

What does the research say for athletic performance?

There are many different types of flavonoids with a wide range of effects. In vitro (test tube) research has shown chrysin is a powerful inhibitor of the aromatase enzyme and may have other health uses.

One thing to remember, is that in vitro research may be misleading when it comes to judging what a compound will do when it's taken orally. That's because the compound in question has to go through the processes of digestion and absorption. It may be changed in the process so that it's inactive, or perhaps even toxic. Or it may never be absorbed at all, but excreted unchanged.

This latter is the most likely outcome. Other bioflavonoids such as quercetin, are notoriously difficult to absorb during digestion and very little gets through. The same may be true for chrysin.

One small study using chrysin containing foods (honey, propolis) showed no effects on serum testosterone after 21 days of feeding.

This study was far from conclusive, as this method of administration was not directly comparable to supplementation. But, another study using human volunteers as well as rats demonstrated that the oral bioavailability of chrysin is low. The researchers stated:

" ...the oral bioavailability of chrysin was estimated to be 0.003–0.02%...Thus the ability of chrysin to influence androgen and oestrogen concentrations in peripheral human target tissues by inhibiting this enzyme is questionable. "

Another study, in which rats were dosed with 50 mg/kg chrysin saw no changes in estrogen or androgen induced uterine growth and came to a similar conclusion.

To date, no solid studies using chrysin in walking, talking, human beings have shown that Chrysin, indeed, can reduce estrogen levels and/or increase testosterone.

What about real world athletic performance?

In truth, I have yet to see anyone who derived any benefit from this supplement.

Will Brink's Recommendation

For reducing estrogen in athletes, chrysin gets a big thumbs down.

References

Gambelunghe C, Rossi R, Sommavilla M, et al. Effects of chrysin on urinary testosterone levels in human males. J Med Food. 2003 Winter;6(4):387-90.

Kellis JT Jr, Vickery LE. Inhibition of human estrogen synthetase (aromatase) by flavones. Science. 1984 Sep 7;225(4666):1032-4.

Pelissero C, Lenczowski MJ, Chinzi D, et al. Effects of flavonoids on aromatase activity, an in vitro study. J Steroid Biochem Mol Biol. 1996 Feb;57(3-4-):215-23.

Saarinen N, Joshi SC, Ahotupa M, et al. No evidence for the in vivo activity of aromatase–inhibiting flavonoids. J Steroid Biochem Mol Biol. 2001 Sep; 78(3):231-9.

Walle T, Otake Y, Brubaker JA, et al. Disposition and metabolism of the flavonoid chrysin in normal volunteers. Br J Clin Pharmacol. 2001 Feb;51(2):143-6.

֎

I3C/DIM

What is it?

Indole–3–carbinol (I3C) is a breakdown product of indole–3–glucosinolate—a compound that is produced in cruciferous vegetables such as cabbage and broccoli. When ingested, I3C is further broken down by stomach acid into diindolylmethane (DIM).

What is it supposed to do?

I3C and DIM are found in certain bodybuilding supplements due to their role as estrogen metabolism modulators. Their role is to induce the formation of "good" estrogen metabolites, which are supposed to compete with testosterone for protein binding, thus enhancing free T while theoretically reducing the negative effects of the "bad" estrogens.

What does the research say for athletic performance?

As alluded to above, not all estrogens are created equal. There are different forms of estrogen in the human body.

Estradiol is the primary form, and can be metabolized in different ways. Certain metabolites, 16–alpha–hydroxyestrone and 4–hydroxyestrone, are thought to be responsible for the carcinogenic effects of estrogen, most notably in breast cancer, but have also been implicated in prostate cancer risk. An alternate metabolic pathway involving the formation of 2–hydroxyestrone, however, carries no such risk. In fact, 2–hydroxyestrone is viewed as being protective against certain cancers, and is known as the "good" estrogen.

A number of in vitro (test tube), rodent, and—now—human studies have demonstrated that indole–3–carbinol, and its metabolites, DIM/ICZ (indolylcarbazole), can influence estrogen metabolism by increasing the formation of 2–hydroxyestrone, and favorably improving the ratio of 2–hydroxyestrone to 16–alpha–hydroxyestrone, a biomarker for cancer risk.

One early study, for example, found that giving 500 mg/day for 1 week to human volunteers, increased estradiol 2–hydroxylation from an average of 29.3% to 45.6%. A later study by the same group demonstrated that intake of I3C (6-7 mg/kg/day) not only increased the urinary excretion of 2–hydroxylated metabolites, but also decreased the amounts of other estrogen metabolites, including estradiol, estrone, estriol, and 16–alpha–hydroxyestrone.

At this point, the evidence in favor of I3C as a possible preventive measure is sufficiently strong, and that clinical trials are being conducted to determine its use for reducing the incidence of breast cancer in women at high risk for developing the disease. DIM may also exert anti-cancer activity directly, by inhibiting the formation of blood vessels that support tumor growth.

So what does this have to do with testosterone? There are a couple of intriguing hypotheses, based on limited evidence. One is an experiment with rats, which showed that injections of estradiol and 4–hydroxyestradiol suppressed LH (luteinizing hormone), while 2–hydroxyestradiol had no effect. A second experiment also showed that administration of 2–hydroxyestradiol immediately before estradiol injection reduced the estradiol–mediated suppression of LH. So it's possible to speculate that I3C/DIM could alter estrogen metabolism in ways that reduce feedback inhibition of testosterone production.

Another hypothesis involves a downstream 2–hydroxylated estrogen metabolite: 2–methoxyestradiol, which has been shown to have an even higher affinity for sex hormone binding globulin (SHBG) than either estradiol or testosterone. It's been speculated that increased levels of 2–methoxyestradiol could compete for SHBG binding and thus increase levels of free T.

Needless to state, there isn't a shred of actual evidence that either of these hypotheses have any merit, or that—even if true—there are any real world benefits for athletes looking to add mass and strength.

What about real world athletic performance?

Indole–3–carbinol in particular is found in several different supplement blends designed to increase T. I've yet to meet anyone who has made any significant gains in mass or strength by using these supplements. The problems are: 1) products sold containing these compounds are very under dosed; and 2) are always mixed with a bunch of other compounds, so useful feedback does not currently exist.

No one to date has taken it alone and in sufficient doses, and had blood work done to see if it was impacting estrogen metabolism and/or T levels.

Will Brink's Recommendation

I3C/DIM may certainly have uses for cancer prevention and/or treatment, and may have legit health uses in general. In theory, it may be a supplement to use with men taking testosterone replacement or athletes using AAS, but that's all hypothetical at this point.

As far as some healthy young guy taking these compounds in hopes of raising T and noticing some actual changes in body composition or strength, forget it. For direct bodybuilding uses (e.g., increased T, increased LBM, increased strength, etc.) I give them two thumbs down at this point.

References

Avvakumov GV, Grishkovskaya I, Muller YA, Hammond GL. Crystal structure of human sex hormone–binding globulin in complex with 2–methoxyestradiol reveals the molecular basis for high affinity interactions with C–2 derivatives of estradiol. J Biol Chem. 2002 Nov 22;277(47):45219-25.

Chang X, Tou JC, Hong C, et al. 3,3'–Diindolylmethane inhibits angiogenesis and the growth of transplantable human breast carcinoma in athymic mice. Carcinogenesis. 2005 Apr;26(4):771-8.

Franks S, MacLusky NJ, Naish SJ, Naftolin F. Actions of catechol oestrogens on concentrations of serum luteinizing hormone in the adult castrated rat: various effects of 4–hydroxyoestradiol and 2–hydroxyoestradiol. J Endocrinol. 1981 May;89(2):289-95.

Michnovicz JJ, Bradlow HL. Induction of estradiol metabolism by dietary indole–3–carbinol in humans. J Natl Cancer Inst. 1990 Jun 6;82(11):947-9.

Michnovicz JJ, Adlercreutz H, Bradlow HL. Changes in levels of urinary estrogen metabolites after oral indole–3–carbinol treatment in humans. J Natl Cancer Inst. 1997 May 21;89(10):718-23.

Muti P, Westerlind K, Wu T, et al. Urinary estrogen metabolites and prostate cancer: a case–control study in the United States. Cancer Causes Control. 2002 Dec;13(10):947-55.

Reed GA, Peterson KS, Smith HJ, et al. A phase I study of indole–3–carbinol in women: tolerability and effects. Cancer Epidemiol Biomarkers Prev. 2005 Aug;14(8):1953-60.

Yuan F, Chen DZ, Liu K, et al. Anti-estrogenic activities of indole–3–carbinol in cervical cells: implication for prevention of cervical cancer. Anticancer Res. 1999 May–Jun;19(3A):1673-80.

℔

6–OXO

What is it?

6–OXO (androst–4–ene–3,6,17–trione) is a naturally occurring compound with anti-aromatase/anti-estrogen properties. It's produced in the human body or can be produced synthetically.

What is it supposed to do?

6–OXO is believed to decrease estrogen and increase testosterone via its effects on the enzyme (aromatase) which converts testosterone to estrogen. 6–OXO appears to be what's known as an irreversible suicide inhibitor of the enzyme.

As the name implies, once bound to the aromatase enzyme, the process cannot be reversed, hence the term "irreversible suicide inhibitor." Translated, 6–OXO binds to the enzyme and prevents it from doing its normal function, which is to produce estrogen from androgens (testosterone, etc.). As most people know, excess estrogen (in particular estradiol) can lead to negative effects such as increased body fat, water retention, gynecomastia (bitch tits), reduced libido, as well as other clinical conditions best avoided. Increased estradiol is often found in steroid users, aging men, as well as other populations.

6–OXO appears to increase testosterone—and keep estrogen in check—by altering a key feedback loop in how the body regulates testosterone production. Exactly how the body regulates various hormones is a very complex topic beyond the scope of this section. Suffice it to say, it primarily involves what's called the hypothalamic-pituitary-testicular axis (HPTA) which works via overlapping negative feedback loops. Estradiol is key in this system. Estradiol is suppressive to testosterone production. High estradiol sends the signal there is high testosterone, and T production is reduced. Lower estrogen, and the body thinks T is low, and sends the signal to produce more T. Reducing estrogen levels is a way to fool the HPTA into producing more T, via an increase in the gonadotropins: follicle stimulating hormone (FSH) and luteinizing hormone (LH)

That's the basic mechanism, which has been greatly over simplified.

The bottom line is: 6–OXO may allow for a more favorable testosterone/estrogen 6–OXO ratio by altering the "set point" for these two hormones. 6–OXO is not an anabolic/androgenic steroid, is not a prohormone, and does not work via androgen receptors or as an anabolic compound directly.

What does the research say for athletic performance?

6–OXO (chemical name androst–4–ene–3,6,17–trione) is also known as 3,6,17–androstenetrione or 6–ketoandrostenedione. In vitro (test tube) and animal studies exist that find 6–OXO acts as a suicide inhibitor of aromatase. That's the good news.

The bad news is, studies in living people are limited. The human studies that exist look quite promising but suffer from a variety of drawbacks, such as the fact they don't appear to have been published in any peer reviewed journals. More on that later.

One study called "The Chronic Effects Of Androst–4–ene–3,6,17–trione On Endocrine Responses In Resistance–trained Men" examined six healthy male subjects, ages 32-40 years of age who were given 300 mg of 6–OXO twice per day for 3 weeks. The study design was open label with 6 participants and ran three weeks.

All subjects followed a specified resistance training program (consisting of 4 days per week) and diet was not controlled for.

The study found total testosterone levels rose an average of 188%, while free testosterone levels rose an average of 226% over the course of the three weeks. The study found there was a slight decrease in estrogen, but the effect was small. They also found no acute toxicity to lipid levels or liver function. The results of this study support the concept of an altered set point for the two hormones vs. a drastic reduction of estrogen.

What about real world athletic performance?

As far as noticing any direct effects on muscle mass or strength, feedback for 6–OXO has been negative with most reporting no changes. However, people that have actually gotten blood work done while using 6–OXO have reported small but consistent increases in testosterone, free testosterone, without an increase in estradiol or a slight decrease.

Will Brink's Recommendation

As anyone can see, the one human study was small (n = 6), short lived, and apparently not published in any journal I am aware of. Taken together with other research (in vitro and animal), 6–OXO is still a compelling supplement in my view. It may be of use for combating issues surrounding elevated estrogen levels due to steroid use, pro hormone use, age, etc.

Recommended dose appears to be 300-600 mg per day. But it's also clear from user feedback that people should not expect any major changes in LBM, body fat, or strength. You should also note that even the small human study mentioned above failed to look at any of those essential outcomes. Clearly, a larger better controlled, and longer study needs to be conducted to get a thumbs up from me.

In theory, an increase in total testosterone, free testosterone, without increases in estradiol, should equal an increase in muscle mass and other positive effects over time, but it's speculation at this time as it applies to 6–OXO. The almost universal negative feedback is puzzling. My hunch is that there needs to be a high enough increase in testosterone to hit some physiological threshold for people to see real changes in body composition.

For example, if one injects 100 mg of testosterone per week (a fairly typical dose for replacement in men with low T), blood work will show a clear increase in this hormone. However, the person will not generally see any changes in body composition. Its not until the person uses at least 200 mg per week (if not more) do we see real changes in body composition, thus there appears to be a threshold that needs to be reached for changes in body composition to occur. Keeping all that in mind, I considered, until it was banned for sale, in the "might be worth a try" category.

However, the issue is now moot as this supplement is no longer legal to sell in the US, although there are batches of it floating around I hear (which is why I left this section in the book) and I recommend people avoid any gray market brands of this supplement.

References

Numazawa M, et al. Mechanism for aromatase inactivation by a suicide substrate, androst–4–ene–3,6,17–trione. The 4 beta, 5 beta–epoxy–19–oxo derivative as a reactive electrophile irreversibly binding to the active site.Biochem Pharmacol. 1996 Oct 25;52(8):1253-9.

Numazawa M, et al. Aromatase inactivation by a suicide substrate, androst–5––ene–4,7,17–trione: the 5beta,6beta–epoxy–19–oxo derivative, as a possible reactive electrophile irreversibly binding to the active site. Biol Pharm Bull. 1997 May;20(5):490-5

Incledon, T. The Chronic Effects Of Androst–4–ene–3,6,17–trione On Endocrine Responses In Resistance–trained Men. Human Performance Specialists, Inc., Chandler, AZ 85249 – tom@thomasincledon.com

℔

Chapter 6

HERBAL TESTOSTERONE BOOSTERS

S hort of seeing an endocrinologist and getting a prescription, there aren't many (legal) ways you can raise testosterone directly via supplements. Yet increasing T has obvious benefits, both for body composition and enhancing libido.

Enter herbal testosterone boosting supplements...

Many plants contain steroidal compounds that are similar in structure to human steroid hormones. Extracts of these plants are consumed in the hope that these compounds will ultimately be converted to testosterone in the body, or else stimulate testosterone production. Not surprisingly, many of the extracts on the market have been used as aphrodisiacs in folk medicine.

Herbal Testosterone Boosters Covered

- ❖ **Avena Sativa**
- ❖ **Fenugreek (Testofen™)**
- ❖ **Horny Goat Weed**
- ❖ **Maca**
- ❖ **Resveratrol**
- ❖ **Tongkat Ali (Long Jack)**
- ❖ **Tribulus Terrestris**
- ❖ **Urtica Dioica**

Herbal supplements are appealing due to the fact that they're "natural"—so presumably safer and more healthy than taking prescription drugs. But, the term "natural" is completely ambiguous and without any science merits. There are lots of things that are completely natural, yet harmful to your health. "Natural" is not synonymous with "safe" or "wholesome." It's a marketing term to be ignored.

Long term health and safety issues aside, the larger question is: do they really work as claimed? Some answers lie in the pages that follow.

AVENA SATIVA

What is it?

Avena sativa is the botanical name for wild oats. The seeds contain various bioactive compounds, such as the alkaloids gramine and avenine; the saponins avenacoside A and B; and avenanthramides, which are polyphenolic compounds with antioxidant activity.

What is it supposed to do?

Avena sativa (AS) has been traditionally used in folk and alternative medicine as a treatment for exhaustion and depression. The reason, however, for its appearance in a growing number of bodybuilding supplements is its reputation as an aphrodisiac and testosterone booster.

What does the research say for athletic performance?

There is certainly plenty of research on oats these days. Oat fiber (especially beta–glucan), for example, can reduce serum cholesterol. As alluded to above, oats also contain antioxidant compounds, known as avenanthramides, that have been shown to have anti-inflammatory and antiatherogenic activity in both animal and in vitro (test tube) experiments. The avenacosides also appear to exert some physiological effects in animal experiments, by increasing intestinal permeability and (slightly) reducing liver lipids.

So where does AS's rep as an aphrodisiac and T-booster come from? Good question.

There isn't a single published study—not even of the aforementioned test tube variety—that suggests wild oats has any effect on either sex hormone levels or libido! There aren't even any reputable unpublished studies, such as conference presentations, posters, etc. As near as I can figure out, AS's reputation comes from one source: an outfit known as "The Institute for Advanced Study of Human Sexuality", based in Northern California. The Institute alleges that their research on the sexually stimulating properties of AS began in 1979, with several research "studies" taking place throughout the 1990s. Not surprisingly, the Institute markets a line of AS supplements under the "Vigorex" label. The Vigorex products are claimed to be homeopathic—which means that the extract has also been extensively diluted. As it says in the glossary, homeopathic preparations are "... an expensive technique for consuming small quantities of water."

The Institute alleges that AS works by increasing the amount of free testosterone. Looking at the text descriptions of the "studies" (which contain no actual data), this claim appears to be based solely on results obtained from 6 subjects, 4 of whom had "... no significant endocrine changes" whatsoever! Suffice it to say, this isn't very convincing. Is there any possibility AS could enhance libido? There is some in vitro (test tube) research that demonstrates avenanthramide–2c can increase nitric oxide (NO) production. In one human feeding study, oats were also shown to enhance endothelial function and vasodilation. The oat alkaloid gramine also has vasorelaxing effects. NO production and vasodilation are important for achieving an erection, so it's possible to speculate that oat compounds could enhance sexual function through this mechanism. But it's a stretch to say that AS supplements actually accomplish this—or accomplish this in the doses seen in bodybuilding supplements.

What about real world athletic performance?

There are very few supplements that are pure AS. I've seen a handful of reviews from users of AS powder, who feel it's been beneficial for mood and sleep. This reaction lends some support to the traditional, medicinal use of oat teas and tonics. I've also seen a couple of positive comments about libido, but this could easily be a placebo effect. Needless to state, not even the few reports I've seen have anything positive to say about increases in strength or lean body mass.

Will Brink's Recommendation

You can guess what I have to say about Avena sativa: it gets a thumbs down from me for increasing muscle or improving performance, let alone increasing T or libido.

References

Bell S, Goldman VM, Bistrian BR, et al. Effect of beta–glucan from oats and yeast on serum lipids. Crit Rev Food Sci Nutr. 1999 Mar;39(2):189-202.

Chen CY, Milbury PE, Kwak HK, et al. Avenanthramides and phenolic acids from oats are bioavailable and act synergistically with vitamin C to enhance hamster and human LDL resistance to oxidation. J Nutr. 2004 Jun;134(6):1459-66.

Froldi G, Silvestrin B, Dorigo P, Caparrotta L. Gramine: a vasorelaxing alkaloid acting on 5–HT(2A) receptors. Planta Med. 2004 Apr;70(4):373-5.

Katz DL, Evans MA, Chan W, et al. Oats, antioxidants and endothelial function in overweight, dyslipidemic adults. J Am Coll Nutr. 2004 Oct;23(5):397-403.

Liu L, Zubik L, Collins FW, et al. The antiatherogenic potential of oat phenolic compounds. Atherosclerosis. 2004 Jul;175(1):39-49.

Nie L, Wise ML, Peterson DM, Meydani M. Avenanthramide, a polyphenol from oats, inhibits vascular smooth muscle cell proliferation and enhances nitric oxide production. Atherosclerosis. 2006 Jun;186(2):260-6.

Onning G, Asp NG. Effect of oat saponins on plasma and liver lipids in gerbils (Meriones unguiculatus) and rats. Br J Nutr. 1995 Feb;73(2):275-86.

Onning G, Wang Q, Westrom BR, et al. Influnce of oat saponins on intestinal permeability in vitro and in vivo in the rat. Br J Nutr. 1996 Jul;76(1):141-51.

☧

FENUGREEK (TESTOFEN™)

What is it?

Fenugreek is Trigonella foenum–graecum L., a medicinal herb also used as a spice and flavoring agent. It's best-known uses are in curry powder and in processed food products where it's used as a maple flavoring.

What is it supposed to do?

Among other traditional medicinal uses, fenugreek is used to treat diabetes, and is sometimes included in OTC diet supplements due to its ability to enhance glycemic control and insulin sensitivity. Its primary use in most bodybuilding supplements, however is as a "natural" way to increase testosterone levels. Testofen™ is a proprietary fenugreek extract used in many current supplements.

What does the research say for athletic performance?

Fenugreek contains a wide range of interesting and potentially useful compounds, including the saponin steroid precursor diosgenin, as well as other saponins, such as yamogenin, gitogenin, smilagenin, and protodioscin. Fenugreek also contains polyphenolic antioxidants as well as an unusual and unique amino acid: 4–hydroxyisoleucine.

There is a fair amount of research on fenugreek as a potential therapeutic agent in diabetes. Both animal studies and a few human studies indicate that fenugreek can help improve glycemic control and reduce the risk of various diabetes related pathologies. In a rat model of diabetes, for example, both water and ethanol extracts of fenugreek seeds significantly reduced blood sugar levels and improved glucose disposition. Oral administration of a water extract of fenugreek seeds to diabetic rabbits for 30 days also significantly lowered fasting blood glucose.

A limited number of human studies have been done, but the results look promising. Fenugreek seed powder (100 g/day) was incorporated into the diets of Type I (insulin dependent) diabetics for 10 days in an Indian clinical study. The researchers concluded that:

" The fenugreek diet significantly reduced fasting blood sugar and improved the glucose tolerance test. There was a 54 per cent reduction in 24-h urinary glucose excretion. Serum total cholesterol, LDL and VLDL cholesterol and triglycerides were also significantly reduced."

A study on Type 2 diabetics receiving 1 g/day of fenugreek seed extract for 2 months had improved glycemic control, reduced insulin resistance and decreased serum triglycerides relative to controls.

Part of fenugreek's ability to improve glucose/insulin status in diabetics is due to 4–hydroxyisoleucine. This unusual amino acid may have some application to athletes: one recent study demonstrated that the addition of 2 mg/kg 4–hydroxyisoleucine to post-workout dextrose improved rates of glycogen resynthesis following a glycogen depletion ride by 63% vs. dextrose alone.

The saponins in fenugreek have been shown to reduce serum cholesterol in animal models. Other experiments have suggested that fenugreek has gastroprotective and hepatoprotective effects. Fenugreek extracts also appear to protect against lipid peroxidation.

What about evidence that fenugreek increases testosterone? The short version is: there isn't any. Not one single study exists that demonstrates that fenugreek has any impact on T levels.

Fenugreek does contain diosgenin, a plant steroid that serves as the raw material for the synthesis of steroids for medical and veterinary use. Mexican wild yam is a principal source of this compound, and wild yam extracts are also sold as supplements to both men and women in the mistaken belief that the diosgenin can be converted to active sex steroids in the body. This is not true, however; the conversion of diosgenin to progesterone, estrogen and/or testosterone can occur only in the laboratory. So people who hope that fenugreek will increase testosterone or have other steroid-like effects due to its diosgenin content are going to be disappointed.

Fenugreek also contains protodioscin, which is presumed to convert to. or stimulate production of, DHEA in the body. Protodioscin is also the active principle in Tribulus terrestris, which is reviewed later in this chapter. As discussed in the review, Tribulus supplementation has no significant effects on either testosterone levels, lean body mass or strength, so it's unlikely that fenugreek would significantly increase T levels due to its protodioscin content either.

That hasn't stopped some supplement companies from trying, however. One company, Gencor Pacific, markets a fenugreek extract called "Testofen™" that appears in certain bodybuilding supplements. Testofen™ is standardized to "50% fenuside" and is claimed to increase testosterone, as well as libido. Gencor Pacific presents selected data from two "in house" rodent studies to back up their claims.

What is "fenuside"? According to the company: "Fenuside is one such saponin glycoside identified by us." Unfortunately, this means that its identity is proprietary information—there is no such compound in the scientific literature.

How does it work? According to the Gencor Pacific's own report: Testofen™ seems to have mode of action through

- The Adrenal Cortex. It seems to stimulate the secretion of Corticotropin Releasing Hormone [CRH] from the Hypothalamus in the brain.

- The CRH reaches the Anterior Pituitary Gland and stimulates it to produce Adrenocorticotropic Hormone [ACTH]. ACTH then acts on the cells of the Adrenal Cortex stimulating them to produce Androgens. Androgens are precursors to Testosterone with Testosterone like activity, the common one being Androstenedione.

It just so happens that the "Androgens" produced from the adrenal cortex are none other than DHEA and—to a lesser extent—androstenediol. It has been well established that this pathway does not contribute significantly to testosterone in men, although it can in women.

This raises the suspicion that maybe "fenuside" is simply protodioscin by another name, although there's no real way to know, short of a laboratory analysis.

And while the limited data Gencor Pacific has available shows an increase in T levels with Testofen™ administration, testosterone increases in mice are alsoseen with DHEA administration. The company has not submitted its studies to any peer reviewed journal, so until an independent test in humans is performed, I remain skeptical of the claims for this extract.

What about real world athletic performance?

Fenugreek and/or Testofen™ are rarely taken "straight", so there's been no relevant feedback on whether or not either have any effect on lean mass or performance. It's safe to say, however, that feedback on the supplements that they're used in has been mixed, at best.

Will Brink's Recommendation

Fenugreek may have benefits to health, and may even be useful to athletes by enhancing post-workout glycogen resynthesis. But for improving strength or building muscle, it gets a thumbs down from me.

References

Broca C, Gross R, Petit P, et al. 4–Hydroxyisoleucine: experimental evidence of its insulinotropic and antidiabetic properties. Am J Physiol. 1999 Oct;277(4 Pt 1):E617-23.

Gupta A, Gupta R, Lal B. Effect of Trigonella foenum–graecum (fenugreek) seeds on glycaemic control and insulin resistance in type 2 diabetes mellitus: a double blind placebo controlled study. J Assoc Physicians India. 2001 Nov;49:1057-61.

Kaviarasan S, Vijayalakshmi K, Anuradha CV. Polyphenol–rich extract of fenugreek seeds protect erythrocytes from oxidative damage. Plant Foods Hum Nutr. 2004 Fall;59(4):143-7.

Muscarella P, Boros LG, Fisher WE, et al. Oral dehydroepiandrosterone inhibits the growth of human pancreatic cancer in nude mice. J Surg Res. 1998 Oct;79(2):154-7.

Puri D, Prabhu KM, Murthy PS. Mechanism of action of a hypoglycemic principle isolated from fenugreek seeds. Indian J Physiol Pharmacol. 2002 Oct; 46(4):457-62.

Ruby BC, Gaskill SE, Slivka D, Harger SG. The addition of fenugreek extract (Trigonella foenum–graecum) to glucose feeding increases muscle glycogen resynthesis after exercise. Amino Acids. 2005 Feb;28(1):71-6.

Sauvaire Y, Ribes G, Baccou JC, et al. Implication of steroid saponins and sapogenins in the hypocholesterolemic effect of fenugreek. Lipids. 1991 Mar; 26(3):191-7.

Sharma RD, Raghuram TC, Rao NS. Effect of fenugreek seeds on blood glucose and serum lipids in type I diabetes. Eur J Clin Nutr. 1990 Apr;44(4):301-6.

Thirunavukkarasu V, Anuradha CV, Viswanathan P. Protective effect of fenugreek (Trigonella foenum graecum) seeds

in experimental ethanol toxicity. Phytother Res. 2003
Aug;17(7):737-43.

Vats V, Grover JK, Rathi SS. Evaluation of anti–hyperglycemic
and hypoglycemic effect of Trigonella foenum–graecum Linn,
Ocimum sanctum Linn and Pterocarpus marsupium Linn in normal
and alloxanized diabetic rats. J Ethnopharmacol. 2002
Jan;79(1):95-100.

⚕

HORNY GOAT WEED

What is it?

Horny Goat Weed is the English version of the Chinese name for herbs of the genus Epimedium: the Chinese yinyanghuo translates to "licentious goat-fire". Legend has it that the name was given by a goat herder who noticed that his goats became more...active after eating the plants. There are 25 known species, although E. grandiflorum, E. sagittatum, E. brevicornum, and E. koreanum appear to be the most widely used and best characterized.

What is it supposed to do?

In traditional Chinese medicine, horny goat weed is used to treat bone fractures and osteoporosis, improve kidney function, treat impotence/infertility and boost the life force or "qi". It's included in a number of bodybuilding supplements as an aphrodisiac and natural testosterone booster.

What does the research say for athletic performance?

Western scientists have shown little interest in horny goat weed research. This deficit has been more than made up for by Chinese researchers, who have conducted extensive research on the herb. The majority of these studies, however, are published in Chinese journals, rather than peer reviewed international journals. So this review is necessarily based on the less extensive work that's been published in more mainstream sources.

As is the case with natural herbal products, horny goat weed has a spectrum of biological activities. One interesting property of the herb is its ability to inhibit bone resorption by osteoclasts in both animal and in vitro (test tube) studies.

Another study found that Epimedium extracts induce osteoblast proliferation. Osteoclasts and osteoblasts are the cells responsible for bone remodeling: osteoblasts build up bone while osteoclasts break it down. So the potential effect of Epimedium in these studies is to preserve and build bone, a function that has possible therapeutic applications for the treatment of osteoporosis.

The major active compound in horny goat weed is thought to be the flavonoid icariin. In vitro studies have shown icariin has potential hepatoprotective, antidepressant and antioxidant activities.

More germane to this review, there is some preliminary evidence that suggests icariin may function as a phosphodiesterase (PDE) inhibitor. Specifically, one in vitro study demonstrated that it inhibits a particular PDE isoform, which is called PDE–5.

Why does this matter? You'll recall from the arginine review, that one of the functions of arginine is the production of nitric oxide, or NO. What NO does when it binds to a receptor is activate the enzyme guanylyl cyclase; which, in turn, manufactures a "second messenger" molecule known as cyclic guanosine monophosphate (cGMP). One of the downstream results of cGMP is the relaxation of vascular smooth muscle. This results in vasodilation and increased blood flow to the surrounding tissues. cGMP is degraded by PDE to 5'–GMP, which has no signalling function. There are 6 different PDE isoforms that occur in different tissues, but they all perform the same basic function.

This is the purpose of using arginine in supplements to boost NO; the idea is to increase NO signalling by making more NO. But there's another way to do it too; by inhibiting the breakdown of cGMP by blocking PDE.

Remember what I said about different PDEs in different tissues? The dominant isoform in the corpus cavernosum is PDE–5. Vasodilation of the corpus cavernosum is what causes an erection. Inhibiting PDE–5 facilitates an erection.

This is how Viagra works: sildenafil citrate is a PDE–5 inhibitor. So the take home from this is that icariin may be a sort of herbal Viagra. There are a few small animal studies that suggest that it also has this activity in vivo, although human studies need to be done. But it at least suggests that icariin, and perhaps horny goat weed, might have some sexual effects.

It is important to remember that Viagra and related compounds for the treatment of erectile dysfunction (ED) do not raise testosterone. T levels were even measured in one of the aforementioned rat studies and the researchers stated:

"Changes in ST [serum testosterone] were not significant".

There is only one study that I found that found icariin had a testosterone-enhancing effect in rats, and the dose was enormous: 200 mg/kg! This is the equivalent of a 20 gram dose in a 100 kg human—of pure icariin, no less. This makes it extremely unlikely that a small dose of horny goat weed extract standardized for icariin will have any impact on T levels.

What about real world athletic performance?

Horny goat weed products get mixed reviews. This may be due to differences in product quality. In a recent Consumer Lab review of different products sold as sexual enhancers, two out of the four horny goat weed extracts tested contained only 31% and 52%, respectively, of the amount of icariin claimed on the label. And the other two products also failed testing due to unacceptably high levels of lead contamination.

Will Brink's Recommendation

Of all of the herbal compounds sold as a libido booster, horny goat weed is possibly the most promising. It is also sold as a T booster, and that does not appear to be the case. People and supplement companies are fixated with testosterone.

If some obscure study comes out showing some animals increased their sexual activity while taking X herb, they immediately start calling it a T booster and assume—versus prove—that's how it must be working.

So far, not one of the herbs that have a reputation as a libido booster (e.g., Tribulus, Long Jack, etc) have been shown to work as T boosters. Thus, just because you see an ad that claims some study found said herb made Sparky the red eyed rodent extra horny does not by any means prove it's a T booster or that it's working through T as a mechanism of action.

There is very little solid information on dose due to the lack of human studies, however, and the quality of the products leave a lot to be desired. Even if it does work, it's not likely to have any significant impact on performance (in the gym, that is) or mass gains.

In my opinion, it may be worth a try for sexual effects, but it gets a thumbs down for boosting T, or increasing mass/strength.

References

Chen KK, Chiu JH. Effect of Epimedium brevicornum Maxim extract on elicitation of penile erection in the rat. Urology. 2006 Mar;67(3):631-5.

Chen KM, Ge BF, Ma HP, et al. Icariin, a flavonoid from the herb Epimedium enhances the osteogenic differentiation of rat primary bone marrow stromal cells. Pharmazie. 2005 Dec;60(12):939-42.

Chiu JH, Chen KK, Chien TM, et al. Epimedium brevicornum Maxim extract relaxes rabbit corpus cavernosum through multitargets on nitric oxide/cyclic guanosine monophosphate signaling pathway. Int J Impot Res. 2006 Jul–Aug;18(4):335-42.

Lee MK, Choi YJ, Sung SH, et al. Antihepatotoxic activity of icariin, a major constituent of Epimedium koreanum. Planta Med. 1995 Dec;61(6):523-6.

Liu WJ, Xin ZC, Xin H, et al. Effects of icariin on erectile function and expression of nitric oxide synthase isoforms in castrated rats. Asian J Androl. 2005 Dec;7(4):381-8.

Liu ZQ. Icariin: a special antioxidant to protect linoleic acid against free–radical–induced peroxidation in micelles. J Phys Chem A Mol Spectrosc Kinet Environ Gen Theory. 2006 May 18;110(19):6372-8.

Meng FH, Li YB, Xiong ZL, et al. Osteoblastic proliferative activity of Epimedium brevicornum Maxim. Phytomedicine. 2005 Mar;12(3):189-93.

Pan Y, Kong L, Xia X, et al. Antidepressant–like effect of icariin and its possible mechanism in mice. Pharmacol Biochem Behav. 2005 Dec;82(4):686-94.

Xin ZC, Kim EK, Lin CS, et al. Effects of icariin on cGMP–specific PDE5 and cAMP–specific PDE4 activities. Asian J Androl. 2003 Mar;5(1):15-8.

Yu S, Chen K, Li S, Zhang K. In vitro and in vivo studies of the effect of a Chinese herb medicine on osteoclastic bone resorption. Chin J Dent Res. 1999 Feb;2(1):7-11.

Zhang ZB, Yang QT. The testosterone mimetic properties of icariin. Asian J Androl. 2006 Sep;8(5):601-5.

 infinity

MACA

What is it?

Maca (Lepidium meyenii) is a root plant native to Peru. It grows at very high altitudes (13,000-14500 ft above sea level) on the Andean plateaus of Peru. It's considered a medicinal food with many uses.

What is it supposed to do?

Maca is similar to ginseng in that it's considered an "adaptogenic" plant based supplement. Like ginseng in Asia, maca has been used for centuries in South America going as far back as 8000 BC during the Inca Empire. The concept of an adaptogen basically means that it helps the body adapt to higher levels of stress.

Unlike ginseng, however, maca is included in bodybuilding supplements due to its alleged aphrodisiac effects.

Maca contains several alkaloids that are said to "nourish" the endocrine glands, including the pituitary, adrenals, pancreas, testes and thyroid gland. Typical of adaptogenic substances, it is believed to have a wide range of effects that include increased strength and performance, increased sexual desire, improved mental acuity, improvements in people with chronic fatigue syndrome, as well as many other effects.

What does the research say for athletic performance?

The above effects are clinical observations in patients rather than the results found in controlled published studies. Unfortunately, there is scant published human research that confirms these clinical observations by doctors in Peru and other parts of the world. There are, however, a few interesting animal studies regarding growth and sexual desire.

One study found that cooked maca, but not raw maca, increased the weights of several generations of mice. They also found the serum values of total proteins and albumin were statistically superior for the mice group eating cooked maca than that of the raw maca and control groups. Does this make maca a true anabolic agent? At least in mice, it appears so but further research is needed.

Another study in rats and mice examined maca's effects on sexual desire and erectile dysfunction. Interestingly, the study found the oral administration of a Maca extract enhanced the sexual function of the mice and rats. The researchers concluded:

"...the present study reveals for the first time an aphrodisiac activity of L. meyenii, an Andean Mountain herb."

Is Maca a true aphrodisiac? Only one small study exists in humans, where doses of 1.5 or 3.0 g/day of maca improved subjective evaluation of sexual desire. But a follow up study by the same researchers in Peru also determined that maca had no effect on testosterone levels. Is it a useful aid to athletes? Unfortunately, these questions can't be definitively answered at this time without better human data to support the animal studies.

What about real world athletic performance?

On a personal note, I tried maca at very high dose (the manufacturer sent me a bunch and asked me to try it) and it did zilch for me. That's an n = 1 observation, so take it for what it's worth. I've heard very little feedback from others.

Will Brink's Recommendation

Maca is a product to keep an eye on and may prove to be a worthwhile supplement to hard training athletes. However, due to its lack of any solid human data, it has to get a thumbs down. Might be worth trying for the heck of it, but I would not get your hopes up too high with this supplement.

References

Canales M, Aguilar J, Prada A, et al. Nutritional evaluation of Lepidium meyenii (MACA) in albino mice and their descendants. Arch Latinoam Nutr. 2000 Jun;50(2):126-33.

Gonzales GF, Cordova A, Vega K, et al. Effect of Lepidium meyenii (MACA) on sexual desire and its absent relationship with serum testosterone levels in adult healthy men. Andrologia. 2002 Dec;34(6):367-72.

Gonzales GF, Cordova A, Vega K, et al. Effect of Lepidium meyenii (Maca), a root with aphrodisiac and fertility–enhancing properties, on serum reproductive hormone levels in adult healthy men. J Endocrinol. 2003 Jan;176(1):163-8.

Zheng BL, He K, Kim CH, et al. Effect of a lipidic extract from lepidium meyenii on sexual behavior in mice and rats. Urology. 2000 Apr;55(4):598-602.

♀

RESVERATROL

What is it?

Resveratrol is 3,5,4'–trihydroxystilbene, an phenolic compound produced by a number of different plants in response to stress. Certain foods, such as grapes and peanuts, contain the highest concentration of resveratrol in the human diet. Red wine is especially rich in resveratrol, containing as much as 13.4 mg/L. Resveratrol is also sold in supplemental form, typically extracted from Polygonum cuspidatum (Japanese Knotweed).

What is it supposed to do?

Resveratrol has a wide range of biological activities. According to a National Institutes of Health summary:

" Health claims of oral dietary supplements containing trans– resveratrol include protection from free-radical damage, inhibition of arthritic inflammation, inhibition of the cyclooxygenase–2 enzyme, protection of blood vessels, protection against cardiovascular disease and cancer, and alleviation of menopausal symptoms. A patent exists for the use of resveratrol to prevent and to treat restenosis after coronary disease treatment, and a patent application was filed for using resveratrol compounds with nucleoside analogs for treating HIV–1 infections."

It's beyond the scope of this review to cover all the possible health effects of resveratrol. Instead, we will confine the discussion to the reasons for its inclusion in this section: its ability to inhibit aromatase and affect estrogen metabolism.

What does the research say for athletic performance?

There is very little human research on the effects of resveratrol. Most of the studies look at the effect of resveratrol consumption from food products, such as red wine. Thus, much of what we know about resveratrol comes from animal and cell culture (test tube) studies.

One recent study on breast cancer cells, showed that resveratrol inhibited aromatase activity and testosterone induced cell proliferation. Resveratrol also acted to reduce the amount of enzyme by reducing the expression of the aromatase mRNA.

One interesting study demonstrated that 20 mg/kg/day of oral trans–resveratrol significantly increased sperm counts in adult male rats. In addition, serum concentrations of FSH (follicle stimulating hormone), LH (luteinizing hormone) and testosterone were significantly higher in the resveratrol treated group. The researchers speculated that—in addition to its ability to inhibit aromatase—resveratrol also functioned as a mixed, weak estrogen receptor agonist/antagonist, but without exhibiting any estrogenic properties. The researchers concluded:

" Our findings indicate that trans–resveratrol merits further research because this phytochemical may constitute a promising new compound for the treatment of male infertility. In Western society, infertility is a growing problem; its causes are diverse, and considerable effort is being made to provide effective therapy. In the case of male infertility, antioxidants, anti–inflammatories, androgens, and antiestrogens are some of the treatments used. However, a truly effective treatment has yet to be found."

On the other hand, a study using a transgenic mouse model for prostate cancer showed no change in serum total testosterone, free testosterone, estradiol, dihydrotestosterone (DHT), and sex hormone binding globulin (SHBG) concentrations in mice given 625 mg resveratrol per kg diet. Resveratrol has been shown to be non-toxic in rats when given 1000 times the amount consumed by a 70-kg person taking 1.4 g of trans-resveratrol/d.

What about real world athletic performance?

Resveratrol is sold as a stand alone supplement, as well as in some anabolic proprietary blends, but I have not had any feedback on resveratrol's ability to increase testosterone at the levels currently found in dietary supplements.

Will Brink's Recommendation

Resveratrol gets a thumb's up from me as a supplement for general health, but we know too little about its effects in humans to recommend it for increasing testosterone or enhancing performance.

References

Hanneke, K. Toxicological Summary for trans–Resveratrol. National Institute of Environmental Health Sciences. March, 2002.

Harper CE, Patel BB, Wang J, et al. Resveratrol Suppresses Prostate Cancer Progression in Transgenic Mice. Carcinogenesis. 2007 Aug 3.

Juan ME, Gonzalez–Pons E, Munuera T, et al. trans–Resveratrol, a natural antioxidant from grapes, increases sperm output in healthy rats. J Nutr. 2005 Apr;135(4):757-60.

Juan ME, Vinardell MP, Planas JM. The daily oral administration of high doses of trans–resveratrol to rats for 28 days is not harmful. J Nutr. 2002 Feb;132(2):257-60.

Wang Y, Lee KW, Chan FL, et al. The red wine polyphenol resveratrol displays bilevel inhibition on aromatase in breast cancer cells. Toxicol Sci. 2006 Jul;92(1):71-7.

 Φ

TONGKAT ALI (LONG JACK)

What is it?

Tongkat Ali (Eurycoma longifolia Jack) also known as Long Jack, is an herb found in Indonesia. It contains compounds known as "quassinoids" such as eurycomalacton, eurycomanon, and eurycomanol as well as others.

What is it supposed to do?

Tongkat Ali (TA) is sold as a male sexual enhancer, muscle builder, and testosterone booster. It has a long history in Indonesia as a male sexual enhancer, with it being sold as a testosterone booster/muscle builder a more recent development.

What does the research say for athletic performance?

Studies in animals showing it increases sexual activity are extensive and compelling. There's many studies that find male rats given TA "do it" more then untreated groups of rats and mice. It seems to work well in young, middle aged, or old rats. Some of those studies are listed below in the reference section. Although interesting, sexual enhancement is not the focus of this book, so I won't take up much space discussing the topic.

The claims of TA being a testosterone booster and muscle builder are what is of interest, and where things get fuzzy from a research perspective. It seems researchers assumed TA was working via increased testosterone in male rats though they don't seem to have actually looked to see if there was an increase in testosterone in these animals, which is odd to say the least and slightly suspicious.

There is mention of paper presented at the "Asian Congress of Sexology" claiming TA increases testosterone in men, but the paper could not be found. It should also be noted that very high doses—between 200 mg/kg to 800 mg/ kg of extract—were used in these studies with rats. The only study that even suggests TA has effects on testosterone and/or works via androgenic pathways examined the effects of TA on the laevator ani muscle in both uncastrated and testosterone stimulated castrated intact male rats. At the highest dose (800 mg/kg) it was found that compared to controls, TA increased the size of this muscle in rats that were both intact and castrated leading the researchers to conclude:

" Hence, the pro–androgenic effect as shown by this study further supported the traditional use of this plant as an aphrodisiac."

Finally, there was an abstract published in the British Journal of Sports Medicine that used real live humans and looked at TA's effects on muscle mass. The results were promising. The study found that 100 mg/kg of TA extract had statistically significant effects on lean body mass, body fat, and strength compared to controls. The study used fourteen men who were put on a strength training program for 5 weeks. The study found the group getting the extract had improved body composition, increased arm circumference, and increased one repetition maximum (1 RM), over the placebo group following the same exercise program. The researchers concluded:

" ...results suggest that water soluble extract of Eurycoma longifolia Jack increased fat free mass, reduced body fat, and increased muscle strength and size, and thus may have an ergogenic effect. Further investigations are warranted."

What about real world athletic performance?

Not much to report for feedback, but most people on my forums report no increases in muscle mass or strength.

Will Brink's Recommendation

The above section on the studies might make one want to run out and buy a case of Long Jack. But wait! There's a bunch of red flags that go up regarding this supplement which should put the breaks on your enthusiasm. For example, the authors in the one study that did use humans and looked at actual changes in LBM and strength states:

" Thus, the objective of this study was to investigate the effect of the increase in testosterone levels, obtained by administration of ELJ, on body composition and muscle strength and size in man. "

All well and fine, so why didn't they actually check their testosterone levels?! Why would one make such a statement then fail to actually look at testosterone levels? Nowhere in the abstract (and it was only published as an abstract vs. as a full paper) do they mention any changes in testosterone, and that's very suspicious. I suspect they did test for testosterone and found no effects, and didn't want to publish that fact, but that's conjecture on my part. All those rat studies, and not one looked at testosterone? Again, something smells fishy…Other big red flags is the fact that if you look at the authors listed in all but one study, they come from essentially one group (Ang and company) from one location: School of Pharmaceutical Sciences, University Science Malaysia, Minden, Penang, Malaysia.

It's not uncommon at all for researchers to attempt to reproduce the effects of another groups findings and fail to get the same results. Anyone remember cold fusion?! HMB also suffered that fate: the people who developed it and had the license for it—which means they made all the money from it—found it was the best thing since anabolic steroids, yet no one else could seem to reproduce the effects. Most of TA's research is published as odd abstracts or papers delivered to places like "the Asian Congress of Sexology." Anyone who has read enough research and knows the basics of research knows a smoke and mirrors group of studies when they see it. This is a shell game that makes TA look impressive "on paper" unless one really looks into it, at which point it's clear something is wrong with the big picture.

Products like this are problematic for me: do I recommend them due to the fact there is a lot of research or do I give it thumbs down because I feel the studies themselves are less then compelling? It's a rock and a hard place for yours truly. Keeping that in mind, due to the amount of research I am going to put TA in the "might be worth a try" category.

However, I make that recommendation with considerable reservation due to the red flags mentioned above. Truth be known, I would not spend my money on it. It may be effective as a male aphrodisiac, but how it works (assuming it works at all) is far from clear at this time and companies selling it as a testosterone booster and muscle builder are full of you-know-what.

References

Ang HH, Cheang HS. Effects of Eurycoma longifolia jack on laevator ani muscle in both uncastrated and testosterone–stimulated castrated intact male rats. Arch Pharm Res. 2001 Oct;24(5):437-40.

Ang HH, Lee KL. Effect of Eurycoma longifolia Jack on libido in middle–aged male rats. J Basic Clin Physiol Pharmacol. 2002;13(3):249-54.

Ang HH, et al. Effects of Eurycoma longifolia Jack on sexual qualities in middle aged male rats. Phytomedicine. 2003;10(6–7):590-3.

Ang HH, et al. Sexual arousal in sexually sluggish old male rats after oral administration of Eurycoma longifolia Jack. J Basic Clin Physiol Pharmacol. 2004;15(3-4):303-9.

Ang HH, Sim MK. Eurycoma longifolia increases sexual motivation in sexually naive male rats. Arch Pharm Res 1998 Dec;21(6):779-81.

Ang HH, et al. Effects of Eurycoma longifolia Jack (Tongkat Ali) on the initiation of sexual performance of inexperienced castrated male rats. Exp Anim. 2000 Jan;49(1):35-8.

Ang HH, Ngai TH. Aphrodisiac evaluation in non–copulator male rats after chronic administration of Eurycoma longifolia Jack. Fundam Clin Pharmacol. 2001 Aug;15(4):265-8.

S. Hamzah, A. Yusof. The ergogenic effects of Eurycoma longifolia jack: a pilot study. Br J Sports Med 2003;37:464-470.

ቀ

TRIBULUS TERRESTRIS

What is it?

Tribulus terrestris is considered a medicinal herb that has been used in many countries as a treatment for impotence and sterility. It's a plant that has been popularized over the years as a possible ergogenic for athletes.

What is it supposed to do?

Supplement companies have claimed it raises testosterone by raising luteinizing hormone (LH). The problem is that we have basically no modern research to go on with healthy athletes. Companies that sell Tribulus often have "in house" research that shows Tribulus raises testosterone but none of this research ever seems to see the light of day in Western peer reviewed medical journals.

What does the research say for athletic performance?

There is in vitro (test tube) research that suggests tribulus may improve the motility, function and total sperm count of animals. And there is some old Bulgarian research with athletes that supposedly showed improvements in strength and performance, but no modern published data showing either increases in testosterone or improvements in performance in athletes. In high enough amounts, some studies have found tribulus to be toxic to animals, but of course many things are toxic at high enough doses that normally present no dangers at lower doses.

At this point, companies marketing tribulus would be better off funding a real study to validate this product as it relates to athletes and testosterone levels, rather than spending the money on advertising.

There was one study in 2000 however, that found some interesting, albeit conflicting, effects with tribulus. Fifteen subjects were randomly assigned to a placebo or tribulus (3.21 mg per kg body weight daily) group.

Body weight, body composition, maximal strength, dietary intake and mood states were determined before and after an 8 week program of periodized weight training and supplementation. The study found there were no changes in body weight, percentage of body fat, total body water, dietary intake or mood states in either group.

Muscle endurance increased for the bench and leg press exercises in the placebo group ($p < .05$; bench press $+/-28.4$ percent, leg press $+/-28.6$ percent), while the tribulus group experienced an increase in leg press strength only (bench press $+/-3.1$ percent, not significant; leg press $+/-28.6$ percent, $p < .05$). According to this study,

" Supplementation with tribulus does not enhance body composition or exercise performance in resistance-trained males."

Why the tribulus group got stronger in the leg press over the placebo group, considering the fact that it had no effects on LBM, fat mass, etc., remains unclear.

A more recent study concluded that supplementation with 10-20 mg/kg body weight (1-2 grams for a 100 kg athlete) had no effect on serum androgen production.

What about real world athletic performance?

Word on the street from users is mixed and this could be due to the quality of the herb, the quantity used, the physical state of the user or the possibility that it just does not work.

Will Brink's Recommendation

Does all this mean tribulus is worthless to athletes? Perhaps not. It does mean that we don't have the kind of evidence we should have before making a recommendation on this supplement.

There is no doubt that as there are many herbs and compounds found within herbs that will turn out to be useful to athletes looking to improve strength, endurance and recuperation from tough workouts. And tribulus may turn out to be one of the herbs, but I would not hold my breath on that one. So, where does this leave us?

Personally, I would be cautious before parting with my money for the stuff. So far, the hype over tribulus far exceeds its worth to athletes. For increasing muscle mass or testosterone levels, tribulus gets a thumbs down at this time.

References

Antonio J, Uelmen J, Rodriguez R, Earnest C. The effects of Tribulus terrestris on body composition and exercise performance in resistance–trained males. Int J Sport Nutr Exerc Metab. 2000 Jun;10(2):208-15.

Bourke CA, Stevens GR, Carrigan MJ. Locomotor effects in sheep of alkaloids identified in Australian Tribulus terrestris. Aust Vet J. 1992 Jul;69(7):163-5.

Miles CO, Wilkins AL, Erasmus GL, Kellerman TS. Photosensitivity in South Africa. VIII. Ovine metabolism of Tribulus terrestris saponins during experimentally induced geeldikkop. Onderstepoort J Vet Res. 1994 Dec;61(4):351-9.

Neychev VK, Mitev VI. The aphrodisiac herb Tribulus terrestris does not influence the androgen production in young men. J Ethnopharmacol. 2005 Oct 3;101(1-3):319-23.

φ

URTICA DIOICA

What is it?

Urtica dioica is commonly known as stinging nettle. It's an edible plant that grows in temperate regions throughout the world. In folk medicine, nettle plants have been used as a diuretic, to treat arthritis, to stimulate lactation and various other uses.

What is it supposed to do?

Stinging nettle contains several lignans that bind to sex hormone binding globulin, or SHBG. SHBG is a glycoprotein that binds to the sex hormones estradiol and testosterone. Bound testosterone is unable to interact with androgen receptors, so theoretically, a compound able to bind SHBG would be able to increase the amount of unbound free T available in the bloodstream.

What does the research say for athletic performance?

Like saw palmetto, stinging nettle is useful for the treatment of benign prostatic hyperplasia (BPH) and associated urinary tract symptoms. In Europe, the two are often combined. One such supplement, "Prostagutt forte"—which consists of 160 mg extract from saw palmetto berries and 120 mg extract from stinging nettle root—produced improvements in men with early stage BPH that were comparable to finasteride (a prescription medication), while producing fewer adverse events.

It is not entirely clear how well stinging nettle works in the absence of saw palmetto. A Brazilian study using 25 mg Pygeum africanum and 300mg stinging nettle extracts found the combination was no more effective than placebo for BPH patients. In vitro (test tube) and rodent studies, however, have made it clear that stinging nettle extracts do have some protective activity against the growth of prostate tissue. It may be that the failure to achieve any results in the Brazilian study was due to differences in the quality of the nettle extracts.

Stinging nettle contains a number of biologically active components. Several Urtica dioica compounds have been found to bind to human sex hormone binding globulin, or SHBG, in vitro. One compound in particular, the lignan (–)–3,4–ivanillyltetrahydrofuran, has a binding affinity described as "outstandingly high" by one research group. (–)–3,4–divanillyltetrahydrofuran has also been shown to interfere with 5 alpha–dihydrotestosterone (DHT) in vitro. Thus, it's possible that there could also be some inhibition in vivo as well, although there is no information on oral bioavailability, what contstitutes a useful dose, what actual effects it might have on the development of lean mass or performance (in the gym or the bedroom), or what side effects might occur. At this point, it's a shot in the dark.

What about real world athletic performance?

There are very few supplements that use either stinging nettle or (–)–3,4–divanillyltetrahydrofuran solo—typically, they are part of various "proprietary blends," which makes it difficult to assess if they have any real effects. Certain supplements containing (–)–3,4–divanillyltetrahydrofuran have gotten good feedback from users, but it's hard to pin down exactly what effects might be attributable to the supplement, and what can be credited to the "placebo effect."

Will Brink's Recommendation

It's impossible to recommend stinging nettle at this time, as there is no evidence that it does anything to increase testosterone or free testosterone, let alone have any effects on LBM or strength. (–)–3,4–divanillyltetrahydrofuran looks promising, but considerably more research needs to be done before I can recommend that either.

References

Melo EA, Bertero EB, Rios LA, Mattos D Jr. Evaluating the efficiency of a combination of Pygeum africanum and stinging nettle (Urtica dioica) extracts in treating benign prostatic hyperplasia (BPH): double–blind, randomized, placebo controlled trial. Int Braz J Urol. 2002 Sep-Oct;28(5):418-25.

Schottner M, Gansser D, Spiteller G. Lignans from the roots of Urtica dioica and their metabolites bind to human sex hormone binding globulin (SHBG).Planta Med. 1997 Dec;63(6):529-32.

Schottner M, Spiteller G, Gansser D. Lignans interfering with 5 alpha–dihydrotestosterone binding to human sex hormone–binding globulin. J Nat Prod. 1998 Jan;61(1):119-21.

Sokeland J. Combined sabal and urtica extract compared with finasteride in men with benign prostatic hyperplasia: analysis of prostate volume and therapeutic outcome. BJU Int. 2000 Sep;86(4):439-42.

φ

Chapter 7

PHYTOCHEMICALS

Higher testosterone levels are good for adding LBM, minimizing body fat, having a healthy libido, etc. but can have negative consequences too. Male pattern baldness, acne, oily skin, and benign prostatic hyperplasia are all potential consequences of increased testosterone due to conversion to DHT. So it's not surprising that there would be a market for compounds that might be anabolic without producing androgenic effects.

Herbal Testosterone Boosters Covered
❖ Beta–Sitosterol
❖ Ecdysterone
❖ Methoxyisoflavone

Herbs produce a vast array of biologically active substances that have been shown to have many different effects. Many function as antioxidants, inhibit the growth of cancer cells, affect neurotransmitter levels, enhance glucose control, reduce inflammation and perform other useful functions. It's conceivable then, that phytochemicals exist that could stimulate muscle protein synthesis or improve performance.

BETA–SITOSTEROL

What is it?

Beta–sitosterol is one of many sterol compounds derived from plants. It has structural similarities to cholesterol, which is produced in the human body and found preformed in various foods. Other sterols derived from plants are campesterol and stigmasterol which are collectively known as phytosterols.

What is it supposed to do?

Beta–sitosterol has a long list of claims, such as immune support, anti-inflammatory effects/pain relief, as a treatment for benign prostate enlargement/benign prostatic hyperplasia, cancer prevention, and as a way to treat high cholesterol levels in humans. In the sports nutrition arena, the claim has been that, due to its structural similarities to cholesterol and other compounds, it builds muscle, since cholesterol is a precursor to anabolic hormones such as testosterone.

Some companies selling this compound claimed that, like cholesterol, it's a precursor for testosterone, while others have claimed it has direct effects beyond conversion to testosterone. Finally, the plant sterol is claimed to prevent the conversion of testosterone to DHT, which is a potent androgen associated with various problems, such as male pattern baldness and prostate enlargement.

What does the research say for athletic performance?

Because the claims for beta–sitosterol (BS) are so varied and the research so extensive, we will stick mostly to the claims germane to this book. Research showing BS improves strength, performance, or muscle mass in humans is essentially non existent.

Interestingly, some studies do suggest high doses of BS fed to animals can alter or increase testosterone production—as well as estrogen (estradiol), which is not necessarily a good thing. However, studies that fed BS to humans didn't find any increase in testosterone.

Other claims for BS are much better supported and compelling. Studies do find it may decrease LDL cholesterol, improve the symptoms of benign prostate enlargement, modulate immune function, reduce the production of inflammatory cytokines, and have anti-cancer effects. For example, animals studies find reductions in tumor growth and reduced metastasis of breast cancer cells when the animals are fed BS. Due to this compelling research on its cholesterol lowering effects, food companies are adding it to margarine and other food stuffs.

More relevant to athletes, data suggests BS may inhibit the post-exercise immune suppression that occurs following intense exercise and possibly suppress the catabolic hormone cortisol. All of these effects mentioned above need further investigation however. A simple reduction in some hormone does not automatically equal increased muscle mass or strength. Many nutrients have been shown to reduce cortisol levels (e.g., vitamin C) yet don't appear to do jack sh*& for muscle mass directly. Research suggests BS is quite safe with no known toxicity.

What about real world athletic performance?

Although I have gotten some positive reports from men using BS for prostate enlargement, no one has ever reported effects such as increased strength, muscle mass, or performance.

Will Brink's Recommendation

BS appears to be one of many compounds found in plant-based foods that have potentially positive health benefits. From an athlete's point of view, the possible effects on cortisol/prevention of post-workout immune suppression may be of interest. However, there is no evidence at all that BS will improve strength, body composition, or performance in any way.

As a testosterone booster, it's a waste of money. As a general health supplement, studies suggest some benefits. Another possible use as it applies to athletes are the studies that suggest SB can block the conversion of testosterone to DHT, and that may have some applications in treating or preventing male pattern baldness and other DHT related issues, but it's far from well researched or proven to have any benefits in this area.

The range of recommended doses is quite wide: from as low as 60 mg to as high as 40 g, with 1–3 g being average. The optimal dose for effects on cholesterol, immunity, or benign prostate enlargement is unclear.

As a general health supplement or as a possible treatment for high cholesterol, BS gets a thumbs up. As a supplement for altering body composition or increasing strength, there are better places to spend your hard earned money.

References

Awad AB, et al. Dietary phytosterol inhibits the growth and metastasis of MDA–MB–231 human breast cancer cells grown in SCID mice. Anticancer Res. 2000 Mar-Apr;20(2A):821-4.

Awad AB, Fink CS. Phytosterols as anticancer dietary components: evidence and mechanism of action. J Nutr. 2000 Sep;130(9):2127-30.

Bouic PJ, Lamprecht JH. Plant sterols and sterolins: a review of their immune–modulating properties. Altern Med Rev. 1999 Jun;4(3):170-7.

Jones PJ, et al. Cholesterol–lowering efficacy of a sitostanol–containing phytosterol mixture with a prudent diet in hyperlipidemic men. Am J Clin Nutr.1999 Jun;69(6):1144-50.

Nieminen P, et al. Phytosterols affect endocrinology and metabolism of the field vole (Microtus agrestis). Exp Biol Med (Maywood). 2003 Feb;228(2):188-93.

Parsons HG, et al. A marked and sustained reduction in LDL sterols by diet and cholestyramine in beta–sitosterolemia. Clin Invest Med. 1995 Oct;18(5):389-400.

Ryokkynen A, et al. Multigenerational exposure to phytosterols in the mouse. Reprod Toxicol. 2005 Mar–Apr;19(4):535-40.

Ⴔ

ECDYSTERONE

What is it?

Ecdysterone is in the phytoecdysteroids family of which there are approximately 200 plant steroids related in structure to the invertebrate steroid hormone 20–hydroxyecdysone.

Though similar in structure as steroids found in humans (i.e. testosterone) close does not cut it in reality. As the saying goes, *"other than horse shoes and hand grenades, close does not count."* What this means is that a steroid hormone has a very specific lock and key fit to its receptor and just because something looks like the same key does not mean it will fit the lock.

What is it supposed to do?

Claims for ecdysterone (beta–ecdysterone) suggest that it may increase protein synthesis in people and has been shown to improve performance in athletes.

What does the research say for athletic performance?

As a rule, western scientists have generally dismissed plant sterols as having any anabolic (muscle building) effects in the human body and consider the sale of such products as a scam and snake oil.

Researchers in places like Japan and Russia have had a much more positive view of Ecdysterone and have come to the conclusion that they do have biological effect in humans and might be useful to athletes. Several Russian scientists I know, and various athletes, swear by certain products whose main ingredient are plant sterols, in particular, ecdysterone.

Though there is little doubt that most plant sterols have no anabolic effects in humans, does that mean all plant sterols have no effects in humans? Did we throw out the baby with the bath water by deciding all plant sterols had no effects in people? It's possible. It has also been shown to increase protein synthesis in some animal models.

But, it should be clearly noted that this research is from the aforementioned countries and has never been confirmed by Western research, which is considered far more stringent. Not to mention the fact that animals are not people.

What about real world athletic performance?

Whatever the value of ecdysterone, the fact remains that very few people taking commercial formulations have seen gains that can be attributed to the supplement. Most supplements contain fairly small doses, however. It's possible that larger amounts might be needed to see an effect.

Will Brink's Recommendation

So what's the bottom line? At this time I see no reason to start running to the store to buy ecdysterone or any other product containing plant sterols for anabolic purposes.

Just know that it might also be wise to not close the door on this topic and be prepared to keep an open mind to the possibilities that some plant sterols, in particular ecdysterone, could be found to have some beneficial effects in humans.

Much more research is needed, however.

Truth be told regarding this writer's feelings on the matter, I would not be holding my breath... For building muscle, ecdysterone gets a thumbs down at this time.

References

Dinan L. Phytoecdysteroids: biological aspects. Phytochemistry. 2001 Jun;57 (3):325-39.

Lafont R, Dinan L. Practical uses for ecdysteroids in mammals including humans: an update. J Insect Sci. 2003;3:7.

Slama K, Koudela K, Tenora J, Mathova A. Insect hormones in vertebrates: anabolic effects of 20–hydroxyecdysone in Japanese quail. Experientia. 1996 Jul 15;52(7):702-6.

Syrov VN. Phytoecdysteroids: their biological effects in the body of higher animals and the outlook for their use in medicine. Eksp Klin Farmakol. 1994 Sep-Oct;57(5):61-6.

Ҩ

METHOXYISOFLAVONE

What is it?

Most people who follow sports nutrition or take supplements intended for the sports nutrition market, have probably heard of methoxyisoflavone (a.k.a. 5–methyl–7–methoxy–isoflavone) or "methoxy" for short. Methoxy is a plant-based compound in the family of compounds known flavanoids, which includes isoflavones, flavones, flavanones, naphthoflavones, as well as others.

This is a very large family of compounds, such as alpha–naphthoflavone, catechin, daidzein, equol, beta–naphthoflavone (BNF), quercetin, rutin, chrysin, genistein, ipriflavone, baicalein, quercetin, galangin, and biochanin.

Amazingly, there are far more of these compounds that I am not even listing! These plant-based compounds have a great range of effects, ranging from anti-cancer, antioxidant, and a thousand other potential uses still being elucidated by researchers as we speak.

What is it supposed to do?

A Hungarian company called Chinoin originally studied methoxy in the 1970s. The company has a patent on methoxy and lists its many effects on metabolism, including increased protein synthesis, increased lean mass, reduced body fat, promoted endurance, lowered cholesterol levels and an improvement in the body's ability to use oxygen.

The patent and supplement companies now selling methoxy claim this plant-based supplement has anabolic effects, working through non-hormonal pathways. That is, it achieves the above without using/affecting hormones such as testosterone, growth hormone, etc. Sound too good to be true? Does to me, too.

What does the research say for athletic performance?

Bodybuilders and other athletes have come to use the term "anabolic" to mean the building of muscle exclusively. This is only partly true. For example, physiology texts book will normally define anabolic or "anabolism" as the phase of metabolism in which simple substances are synthesized into the complex materials of living tissue or a process by which larger molecules are formed from smaller ones.

What does this mean to the reader in English? It means that making new bone, or even fat, is in fact technically an anabolic endeavor. Several companies have done research with isoflavones and found they may increase bone mass in animals and people. Does this mean methoxy affects bone and not muscle? Well, there is very little research with methoxy on healthy active adults that looked at muscle mass, other than the old Hungarian research, so it's hard to tell right now.

Several isoflavones, including methoxy, have been shown to increase the weight of many animals, but again, that effect appeared to be mostly increases in bone density. It should be noted that there is a great deal of research going on right now with hundreds of different plant-based compounds and the flavanoids are perhaps some of the most interesting and promising. But, at this time, methoxy is far from the wonder anabolic supplement as it's being portrayed.

What about real world athletic performance?

I have yet to meet anyone who's achieved any gains in LBM from the simple addition of methoxy. A few have claimed good results from using methoxy supplements, but these people are inevitably stacking multiple compounds and it's impossible to tell whether the results were actually obtained from using the supplement.

Will Brink's Recommendation

Is methoxy a waste of money? Perhaps not, but its exact role in sports nutrition remains unclear, at best. Considering the total lack of data showing any effects on muscle mass of healthy athletes, methoxy gets a thumbs down at this time.

References

Feuer L, Nogradi M, Gottsegen A, Vermes B, et al. Anabolic–weight–gain promoting compositions containing isoflavone derivatives and method using same. United States Patent 3,949,085. 1976 Apr 6.

Feuer L, Farkas L, Nogradi M, Vermes B, et al. Metabolic 5–methyl–isoflavone–derivatives, process for the preparation thereof and compositions containing the same. United States Patent 4,163,746. 1979 Aug 7.

☦

Chapter

8

ADAPTOGENS

A daptogens are compounds extracted from plant sources that improve resistance to stress. Resistance exercise imposes considerable physical stress that requires a certain amount of rest and recovery to avoid overtraining and injury. Everyday life also imposes a certain amount of mental and physical stress, that can take a toll on recovery.

Adaptogens Covered

❖ Ashwagandha

❖ Bacopa Monnieri

❖ Cordyceps

❖ Ginseng

❖ Rhodiola Rosea

Excessive stress can lead to overproduction of catabolic hormones like cortisol, depressed immunity, and poor performance. There are potential benefits then, to supplementing with compounds that might improve recovery or the ability to cope with increased stress.

The adaptogenic compounds on the market today are a part of traditional folk medicine in countries like China, Korea, and Russia. Several have been researched for use by Russian athletes, but have not been extensively evaluated by Western peer reviewed research.

ASHWAGANDHA

What is it?

Ashwagandha is Withania somnifera, a medicinal plant used in traditional Ayurvedic medicine. The name means "smells like a horse", because of the characteristic odor. It's also known as "Indian Ginseng" although it is not related to true ginseng.

What is it supposed to do?

Ashwagandha is used to treat a variety of ailments in Ayurvedic medicine. In bodybuilding supplements, extracts of Withania are supposed to improve stamina and reduce cortisol levels. Ashwagandha is also found in "thyroid support" formulas.

What does the research say for athletic performance?

Most of the studies on Ashwagandha have been performed in rats and mice. In one study, for example, administration of 2.5 mg/kg of an isolated "Withanolide" compound, 1–oxo–5beta, 6beta–epoxy–witha–2–ene–27–ethoxy–olide, resulted in reduced indices of stress from exposure to cold, hypoxia, and restraint. Another study found that the stress–related responses (glucose intolerance, increase in plasma corticosterone levels, gastric ulcerations, male sexual dysfunction, etc.) of rats exposed to random foot shocks were attenuated by 25-50 mg/kg doses of Withania, administered 1 hour before.

Ashwagandha may also have anti-depressant effects. One study demonstrated that daily doses of 20 and 50 mg/kg of the withanolide fraction had similar effects to the benzodiazepine drug lorazepam on rat behavior in "elevated plus-maze, social interaction and feeding latency in an unfamiliar environment" tests.

Some of its positive effects may be due to its antioxidant activity. Rats given injections of 10-20 mg/kg of glycowithanolides for 21 days, had increased levels of endogenous antioxidants (superoxide dismutase, catalase and glutathione Ashwagandha peroxidase) in their brains.

There are also antimicrobial, antiosteoporotic, antitumor, neuroprotective and immune-stimulating properties. Feeding 0.75-1.5 g/day of the root powder to rats also reduced cholesterol in hypercholesterolemic rats.

One of the more interesting properties of Ashwagandha may be its ability to increase levels of thyroid hormones. Mice gavaged with 1.4 g/kg root extract for 20 days had increased serum levels of T3 and T4, along with reduced hepatic lipid peroxidation.

There is even a case report of thyrotoxicosis in a woman taking a supplement containing Ashwagandha. As I've often pointed out, rats and mice aren't people. While these studies look interesting and support the traditional use of the herb, they're far from conclusive.

There are very few human studies that provide any indication of benefits to health or performance at doses normally found in bodybuilding supplements. One of the few human studies involved an Indian commercial supplement, RA-11, which is used to treat arthritis. The 32 week trial demonstrated significantly reduced pain and increased knee function in patients receiving the supplement vs. those receiving the placebo. One flaw, however, was that RA-11 contains several other herbs in addition to Ashwagandha, so it's difficult to draw firm conclusions from this clinical trial.

What about real world athletic performance?

Feedback on this herb has been limited, but mildly positive. There don't appear to be any real benefits to performance, although some users report feeling a greater sense of well-being and/or improved memory.

Will Brink's Recommendation

On paper, Ashwagandha seems like interesting stuff, but it may be that the limited amounts consumed in many commercial supplements are inadequate to produce any real results. Or it could be simply that the rat studies simply don't extrapolate well to people.

In general, this herb is not expensive, so it might be worth a try for overall mood and/or cognition, although it gets a thumbs down for lean mass/performance. It appears to be fairly safe when taken in recommended doses (3-6 g/day of the dried root, or 300-500 mg of a standardized extract). There are potential GI symptoms in higher doses, not to mention the case report of thyrotoxicosis mentioned above.

References

Ahmad M, Saleem S, Ahmad AS, et al. Neuroprotective effects of Withania somnifera on 6–hydroxydopamine induced Parkinsonism in rats. Hum Exp Toxicol. 2005 Mar;24(3):137-47.

Bhattacharya SK, Muruganandam AV. Adaptogenic activity of Withania somnifera: an experimental study using a rat model of chronic stress. Pharmacol Biochem Behav. 2003 Jun;75(3):547-55.

Bhattacharya SK, Bhattacharya A, Sairam K, et al. Anxiolytic–antidepressant activity of Withania somnifera glycowithanolides: an experimental study. Phytomedicine. 2000 Dec;7(6):463-9.

Bhattacharya SK, Satyan KS, Ghosal S. Antioxidant activity of glycowithanolides from Withania somnifera. Indian J Exp Biol. 1997 Mar;35(3):236-9.

Chopra A, Lavin P, Patwardhan B, Chitre D. A 32-Week Randomized, Placebo–Controlled Clinical Evaluation of RA–11, an Ayurvedic Drug, on Osteoarthritis of the Knees. J Clin Rheumatol. 2004 Oct;10(5):236-245.

Girish KS, Machiah KD, Ushanandini S, et al. Antimicrobial properties of a non-toxic glycoprotein (WSG) from Withania somnifera (Ashwagandha). J Basic Microbiol. 2006;46(5):365-74.

Khan B, Ahmad SF, Bani S, et al. Augmentation and proliferation of T lymphocytes and Th–1 cytokines by Withania somnifera in stressed mice. Int Immunopharmacol. 2006 Sep;6(9):1394-403.

Kaur P, Sharma M, Mathur S, et al. Effect of 1–oxo–5beta, 6beta–epoxy–witha–2–ene–27–ethoxy–olide isolated from the roots of Withania somnifera on stress indices in Wistar rats. J Altern Complement Med. 2003 Dec;9(6):897-907.

Mohan R, Hammers HJ, Bargagna–Mohan P, et al. Withaferin A is a potent inhibitor of angiogenesis. Angiogenesis. 2004;7(2):115-22.

Monograph. Withania somnifera. Altern Med Rev. 2004 Jun;9(2):211-4.

Nagareddy PR, Lakshmana M. Withania somnifera improves bone calcification in calcium-deficient ovariectomized rats. J Pharm Pharmacol. 2006 Apr;58(4):513-9.

van der Hooft CS, Hoekstra A, Winter A, et al. Thyrotoxicosis following the use of ashwagandha. Ned Tijdschr Geneeskd. 2005 Nov 19;149(47):2637-8.

Visavadiya NP, Narasimhacharya AV. Hypocholesteremic and antioxidant effects of Withania somnifera (Dunal) in hypercholesteremic rats. Phytomedicine. 2006 May 16.

ቀ

BACOPA MONNIERI

What is it?

Bacopa monnieri is another Ayurvedic medicinal herb, traditionally known as "Brahmi." It's been used for several centuries to treat anxiety and depression, as well as enhance cognition and memory. A number of biologically active compounds have been identified, and are known collectively as "bacosides."

What is it supposed to do?

Bacopa extracts are added to bodybuilding supplements to decrease mental fatigue and assist recovery due to the herb's reputed anti-stress and known antioxidant activities.

What does the research say for athletic performance?

As with Ashwagandha, there is a fair amount of research on the properties and activities of Bacopa monnieri. Unfortunately, most of the work has been done using either rodent or in vitro (test tube) models. What there is, however, makes it clear that Bacopa contains some interesting and pharmacologically active compounds.

One study on rats, for example, demonstrated that pretreatment with 80 mg/kg of a standardized Bacopa extract reduced the physiological changes associated with both acute (1 day) and chronic (7 day) immobilization stress. Another rat study demonstrated that doses of 20 and 40 mg/kg bacosides for 7 days prior to stress altered the expression or activities of certain enzymes in their brains.

The researchers hypothesized that the alterations might allow

"... the brain to be prepared to act under adverse conditions."

Other studies on memory and cognition have demonstrated that Bacopa monnieri may help prevent dementia. A study in mice showed it improved learning following treatment with scopolamine, while another had similar results following treatment with phenytoin. A recent study found that doses of either 40 or 160 mg/kg/day of Bacopa extract reduced the formation of amyloid plaques Bacopa monnieri in a mouse model of Alzheimer's Disease.

Some human studies have also been conducted. An Australian test showed that chronic use of a "Brahmi" preparation on 76 adults between 40 and 65 years of age showed "... a significant effect of the Brahmi on a test for the retention of new information."

A similar conclusion was reached by a different group of researchers who gave their test subjects a daily dose of 300 mg/kg Bacopa extract for 12 weeks. They wrote:

" B. monniera significantly improved speed of visual information processing measured by the IT task, learning rate and memory consolidation measured by the AVLT (P<0.05), and state anxiety (P<0.001) compared to placebo, with maximal effects evident after 12 weeks...These findings suggest that B. monniera may improve higher order cognitive processes that are critically dependent on the input of information from our environment such as learning and memory."

On the other hand, a study using a commercial supplement containing 300mg Bacopa extract and 120 mg Gingko biloba for 4 weeks concluded that the extracts:

" ... did not demonstrate any significant effects on tests investigating a range of cognitive processes including attention, short–term and working memory, verbal learning, memory consolidation, executive processes, planning and problem solving, information processing speed, motor responsiveness and decision making."

Why the difference? It may be due to the quality of the extracts in commercial formulations. One recent analysis found that:

" The total saponin content in the samples, plant materials and extracts varied from 5.1 to 22.17% and 1.47 to 66.03 mg/capsule or tablet in the commercial formulations."

Several other animal studies have also found Bacopa extracts possess antioxidant, anti-inflammatory, hepatoprotective, gastroprotective and neuroprotective effects. A high dose of 200 mg/kg also increased thyroid (T4) hormone levels in mice.

What about real world athletic performance?

A few reviews I've seen for certain standardized Bacopa extracts suggests it has a relaxing quality. Some feel it helps with anxiety. This is in line with its traditional use. There is no indication, however, that it helps w/physical performance.

Will Brink's Recommendation

Bacopa seems to have more nootropic than performance effects. It may be worth a try for people interested in that sort of thing, although there are probably better supplements to take for concentration and focus in the gym. For those who are interested, a recommended dose is 200-400 mg for an extract that is standardized to 20% bacosides.

References

Chowdhuri DK, Parmar D, Kakkar P, et al. Antistress effects of bacosides of Bacopa monnieri: modulation of Hsp70 expression, superoxide dismutase and cytochrome P450 activity in rat brain. Phytother Res. 2002 Nov;16(7):639-45.

Das A, Shanker G, Nath C, et al. A comparative study in rodents of standardized extracts of Bacopa monniera and Ginkgo biloba: anticholinesterase and cognitive enhancing activities. Pharmacol Biochem Behav. 2002 Nov;73(4):893-900.

Holcomb LA, Dhanasekaran M, Hitt AR, et al. Bacopa monniera extract reduces amyloid levels in PSAPP mice. J Alzheimers Dis. 2006 Aug;9(3):243-51.

Kar A, Panda S, Bharti S. Relative efficacy of three medicinal plant extracts in the alteration of thyroid hormone concentrations in male mice. J Ethnopharmacol. 2002 Jul;81(2):281-5.

Monograph: Bacopa monniera. Altern Med Rev. 2004 Mar;9(1):79-85.

Murthy PB, Raju VR, Ramakrisana T, et al. Estimation of Twelve Bacopa Saponins in Bacopa monnieri Extracts and Formulations by High–Performance Liquid Chromatography. Chem Pharm Bull (Tokyo). 2006 Jun;54(6):907-11.

Nathan PJ, Tanner S, Lloyd J, et al. Effects of a combined extract of Ginkgo biloba and Bacopa monniera on cognitive function in healthy humans. Hum Psychopharmacol. 2004 Mar;19(2):91-6.

Rai D, Bhatia G, Palit G, et al. Adaptogenic effect of Bacopa monniera (Brahmi). Pharmacol Biochem Behav. 2003 Jul;75(4):823-30.

Rohini G, Sabitha KE, Devi CS. et al. Bacopa monniera Linn. extract modulates antioxidant and marker enzyme status in fibrosarcoma bearing rats. Indian J Exp Biol. 2004 Aug;42(8):776-80.

Roodenrys S, Booth D, Bulzomi S, et al. Chronic effects of Brahmi (Bacopa monnieri) on human memory. Neuropsychopharmacology. 2002 Aug;27(2): 279-81.

Vohora D, Pal SN, Pillai KK. Protection from phenytoin-induced cognitive deficit by Bacopa monniera, a reputed Indian nootropic plant. J Ethnopharmacol. 2000 Aug;71(3):383-90.

ॐ

CORDYCEPS

What is it?

Cordyceps is a genus of fungi that are classified as "entomopathogenic"—that is, they parasitize and grow on insects, eventually killing them. The most famous of the genus is Cordyceps sinensis, which grows on caterpillars found in southwest China and Tibet. These "vegetable caterpillars" are prized for their health–giving properties, and hold a hallowed place in traditional Chinese medicine. Most of the Cordyceps used in commercial supplements, however, is grown by fermentation in liquid culture media–not on bugs!

What is it supposed to do?

Cordyceps became known to the West after Chinese track and field athletes set several new world records in the early 1990s and attributed their success to it. Cordyceps is touted as an adaptogen, and is claimed to increase stamina and "vital energy." Several active compounds have been identified, including cordycepin and cordycepic acid.

What does the research say for athletic performance?

Much of the research on Cordyceps has been done in China, although some mainstream Western research has been performed as well. The studies indicate that Cordyceps has some genuine biological activity. For example, several studies have demonstrated that Cordyceps has antioxidant activity, and can inhibit lipid peroxidation. In addition, two studies in rats demonstrated enhanced glucose disposal and increased insulin sensitivity after consumption of a commercial Cordyceps supplement. One study in pigs even demonstrated improved sperm quality and quantity after supplementation with the mycelia from Cordyceps militaris.

Some studies have shown that Cordyceps may enhance immunity too. In one experiment, a compound isolated from Cordyceps inhibited the progression of certain symptoms in a mouse model of lupus (an autoimmune disease). Other experiments have shown enhancements in immune cell proliferation andmodulate cytokine production.

One problem, however, with in vitro (test tube) and rodent experiments is dose—typically, the doses used in these types of experiments are much higher than those used in over-the-counter supplements. Thus, many promising compounds may be less effective in humans. Unfortunately, there isn't a lot of research on the effects of Cordyceps on human health. In one small pilot study conducted by Dr. Paul Greenhaff, 18 healthy adults were given 3 x 1 g Cordyceps/day for 4 weeks. Blood/serum chemistries, resting heart rate and blood pressure, respiratory function, and grip strength/endurance were measured at times 0, 2 weeks and 4 weeks. At the end of the study, Dr. Greenhaff concluded:

" There was no demonstrative impact on both metabolic nor physiological measurements with the application of Cordyceps sinensis supplementation in the eighteen healthy subjects. At the same time, there were no side–effects noted or recorded by the subjects. "

Nor has Cordyceps had any impact on human exercise performance—at least endurance performance. Three grams per day of a commercial Cordyceps supplement had no effect on aerobic capacity or endurance exercise performance in endurance–trained male cyclists. A combination of Cordyceps and Rhodiola did not improve muscle tissue oxygen saturation in male subjects during maximal exercise.

What about real world athletic performance?

Feedback from users of this supplement has actually been pretty positive, with people reporting increased energy, "feelings of well-being" and greater energy in the gym, so it may still be worth a try. Doses tend to vary a great deal due to the fact that extracts differ in their concentration of active ingredients. Generally speaking, recommended doses have been between 1 and 4 grams per day, with a dose somewhere in the middle being common.

Will Brink's Recommendation

If you should decide to try Cordyceps, look for a product that is standardized to 5-7% cordycepic acid. Start at 1 g and work your way up to 4 g and see if you notice any improvements in the gym. So far, this supplement is not associated with any significant side effects.

References

Balon TW, Jasman AP, Zhu JS. A fermentation product of Cordyceps sinensis increases whole-body insulin sensitivity in rats. J Altern Complement Med. 2002 Jun;8(3):315-23.

Colson SN, Wyatt FB, Johnston DL, et al. Cordyceps sinensis– and Rhodiola rosea–based supplementation in male cyclists and its effect on muscle tissue oxygen saturation. J Strength Cond Res. 2005 May;19(2):358-63.

Greenhaff, Paul L. Pilot Study to Investigate the Changes in Metabolic and Physiological Parameters using Cordyceps sinensis supplementation (3 grams per day) in a double blind, randomized format (downloaded from http://mycologyresearch.com/pdf/articles/Paul_Leonard_Greenhaff.pdf)

Koh JH, Yu KW, Suh HJ, et al. Activation of macrophages and the intestinal immune system by an orally administered decoction from cultured mycelia of Cordyceps sinensis. Biosci Biotechnol Biochem. 2002 Feb;66(2):407-11.

Li SP, Li P, Dong TT, Tsim KW. Anti–oxidation activity of different types of natural Cordyceps sinensis and cultured Cordyceps mycelia. Phytomedicine. 2001 May;8(3):207-12.

Lin WH, Tsai MT, Chen YS, et al. Improvement of Sperm Production in Subfertile Boars by Cordyceps militaris Supplement. Am J Chin Med. 2007;35(4):631-41.

Parcell AC, Smith JM, Schulthies SS, et al. Cordyceps Sinensis (CordyMax Cs–4) supplementation does not improve endurance exercise performance. Int J Sport Nutr Exerc Metab. 2004 Apr;14(2):236-42.

Wu Y, Sun H, Qin F, Pan Y, Sun C. Effect of various extracts and a polysaccharide from the edible mycelia of Cordyceps sinensis on cellular and humoral immune response against ovalbumin in mice. Phytother Res. 2006 Aug;20(8):646-52.

Yamaguchi Y, Kagota S, Nakamura K, et.al. Inhibitory effects of water extracts from fruiting bodies of cultured Cordyceps sinensis on raised serum lipid peroxide levels and aortic cholesterol deposition in atherosclerotic mice. Phytother Res. 2000 Dec;14(8):650-2.

Yamaguchi Y, Kagota S, Nakamura K, et al. Antioxidant activity of the extracts from fruiting bodies of cultured Cordyceps sinensis. Phytother Res. 2000 Dec;14(8):647-9.

Yang LY, Chen A, Kuo YC, Lin CY. Efficacy of a pure compound H1–A extracted from Cordyceps sinensis on autoimmune disease of MRL lpr/lpr mice. J Lab Clin Med. 1999 Nov;134(5):492-500.

Zhao CS, Yin WT, Wang JY, et al. CordyMax Cs–4 improves glucose metabolism and increases insulin sensitivity in normal rats. J Altern Complement Med. 2002 Jun;8(3):309-14.

☦

GINSENG

What is it?

Ginseng is the dried root of several different species of herbs in the Panax genus. Chinese or Asian Ginseng is Panax ginseng; while American Ginseng is Panax quinquefolius L. Siberian or Russian Ginseng is actually a different, distantly related plant, Eleutherococcus senticosus, and contains different active compounds. Any or all of these might be included in commercial ginseng supplements.

What is it supposed to do?

Ginseng has been used in the Orient for centuries as an "adaptogenic" plant based supplement. The concept of an adaptogen basically means that it helps the body adapt to higher levels of stress. The ailments Ginseng is claimed to treat range from nervous disorders, anemia, poor libido, wakefulness, forgetfulness and confusion, nausea, chronic fatigue, and angina, to name a few.

What does the research say for athletic performance?

Exactly how ginseng supposedly accomplishes all this is unclear and still being investigated. In animals, ginseng appears to have positive effects on the cardiovascular system, central nervous system, endocrine system, metabolism, and immune system. However, several recent reviews that examined the data on ginseng concluded, that while studies with animals show that ginseng (or its active components) may have positive effects on health and performance, there is generally a lack of controlled research demonstrating the ability of ginseng to improve performance in humans.

The general consensus regarding the effects of ginseng in humans is that most studies suffer from methodological problems such as inadequate sample size and lack of double blind, control and placebo designs. However, Germany's Commission E, which is responsible for developing guidelines for herbs, has found that ginseng is useful for a wide variety of problems, such as fatigue and improving mental concentration. Europeans seem to have a much better handle on the uses of ginseng than the US.

To the reader, the above may seem confusing or contradictory. The reason for the contradictory information may be due in part to the type of ginseng being used, the quality of the ginseng being used, the amount of the ginseng used, and the aforementioned study design problems. For example, different varieties of ginseng are reported to have different effects.

Also, many ginsengs on the market are known to be lacking in the active ingredients. In true ginseng these are known as "ginsenosides"; similarly, the active compounds in Siberian Ginseng are known as "eleutherosides". One study found that over 85 percent of ginseng products on the shelves contained virtually no ginsenosides. This makes ginseng something of a confusing supplement for athletes, but not a supplement without potential merit. One recent study, for example, found 350 mg of ginseng extract improved the reaction time (psychomotor performance) of soccer players over a six week period.

Overall, studies on ginseng and athletic performance have yielded mixed results, with some studies showing modest improvements in endurance and time to exhaustion, while others show no effect.

Some studies have found ginseng has powerful anti-cancer and antioxidant properties, as well as an ability to improve blood sugar metabolism. One recent study found ginseng was able to treat some men with erectile dysfunction!

This may be due to ginseng being possibly able to effect nitric Oxide (NO) production in men, as NO is essential for obtaining an erection.

What about real world athletic performance?

By some accounts with users, various ginseng preparations seem to increase stamina, concentration and resistance to stress, as well as improvements in endurance. Others report no discernable effects.

Will Brink's Recommendation

The use of ginseng continues to grow with current sales estimated to be approximately 300 million dollars annually. There is clearly a need for research dealing with the efficacy of ginseng. This research needs to take into account basic, fundamental design considerations if there is to be any hope of establishing whether or not ginseng actually has a place in an athlete's supplement regimen. It's hard to imagine a billion Chinese could be totally wrong about ginseng however...

What is the optimal dose? Different extracts contain differing amounts of the active ingredients. Different products contain different doses. General recommendations are commonly 50-100 mg per day of an extract containing at least 7 percent-10 percent ginsenosides, 2-3 times per day.

Some experimentation may be needed however. What about building muscle? There is not a drop of solid data to support such a use for ginseng. So, an athlete looking to build muscle or increase performance, ginseng gets a thumbs down.

References

Bahrke MS, Morgan WP. Evaluation of the ergogenic properties of ginseng. Sports Med. 1994 Oct;18(4):229-48.

Bahrke MS, Morgan WR. Evaluation of the ergogenic properties of ginseng: an update. Sports Med. 2000 Feb;29(2):113-33.

Ong YC, Yong EL. Panax (ginseng)—panacea or placebo? Molecular and cellular basis of its pharmacological activity. Ann Acad Med Singapore. 2000 Jan;29(1):42-6.

Sotaniemi EA, Haapakoski E, Rautio A. Ginseng therapy in non–insulin–dependent diabetic patients. Diabetes Care. 1995 Oct;18(10):1373-5.

Vogler BK, Pittler MH, Ernst E. The efficacy of ginseng. A systematic review of randomised clinical trials. Eur J Clin Pharmacol. 1999 Oct;55(8):567-75.

Ziemba AW, Chmura J, Kaciuba–Uscilko H, et al. Ginseng treatment improves psychomotor performance at rest and during graded exercise in young athletes. Int J Sport Nutr. 1999 Dec;9(4):371-7.

℔

RHODIOLA ROSEA

What is it?

Rhodiola rosea is a popular traditional medicinal plant in Eastern Europe and Asia. It contains a number of biologically active compounds, which include salidroside, p–tyrosol, and what are collectively known as "rosavins".

What is it supposed to do?

Rhodiola preparations have been used to reduce fatigue, prevent high-altitude sickness, and treat depression. Rhodiola extracts in bodybuilding supplements are supposed to reduce the effects of stress and enhance recovery.

What does the research say for athletic performance?

Rhodiola rosea has been extensively researched in Eastern Europe. Unfortunately, much of the work has been published in obscure (mostly) Russian language journals and has not been evaluated by the standards of Western, peer reviewed science.

One study published in the International Journal of Sports Nutrition and Exercise Metabolism found that acute intake of 200 mg Rhodiola extract standardized for 3% rosavins and 1% salidroside modestly increased the endurance exercise capacity in young, healthy volunteers.

Other studies have shown limited, but positive results. One study using simulated high-altitude conditions showed that supplementation with Rhodiola extract tended to decrease the formation of free radicals produced under hypoxic stress. A second study demonstrated an anti-inflammatory effect in the muscles of untrained volunteers participating in exhaustive exercise.

Other human studies, however, have shown no effects on performance. Two studies using commercial supplements containing Rhodiola extracts as a part of a blend showed no significant impact on cycling performance.

Animal studies suggest that Rhodiola rosea possesses possible adaptogenic activity. One study in mice showed that a standardized extract (3% rosavins, 1% salidroside) had adaptogenic, antidepressant and stimulating effects when given at doses ranging from 10-20 mg/kg. Another found that 50 mg/kg Rhodiola extract increased the time to exhaustion of swimming rats.

Rhodiola extracts have been found to improve glycemia and increase the levels of endogenous antioxidant enzymes in the livers of diabetic rats.

Other interesting properties have emerged from in vitro (test tube) work. Rhodiola extracts may have some anti-hypertensive, anti-tumor, and antimicrobial effects.

What about real world athletic performance?

User feedback has been generally positive for extracts that have been standardized for 3% rosavins. People who use it feel it seems to help with overall mood and reduction of fatigue.

Will Brink's Recommendation

Rhodiola does not appear to be much of a performance-enhancer, although I suppose it might be "worth a try" for overall resistance to fatigue. If you should decide to try it, look for a supplement that provides at least 100-200 mg of an extract standardized to 3% rosavins.

References

Abidov M, Grachev S, Seifulla RD, Ziegenfuss TN. Extract of Rhodiola rosea radix reduces the level of C–reactive protein and creatinine kinase in the blood. Bull Exp Biol Med. 2004 Jul;138(1):63-4.

Abidov M, Crendal F, Grachev S, et al. Effect of extracts from Rhodiola rosea Chapter 5/Rhodiola rosea and Rhodiola crenulata (Crassulaceae) roots on ATP content in mitochondria of skeletal muscles. Bull Exp Biol Med. 2003 Dec;136(6):585-7.

Colson SN, Wyatt FB, Johnston DL, et al. Cordyceps sinensis– and Rhodiola rosea–based supplementation in male cyclists and its effect on muscle tissue oxygen saturation. J Strength Cond Res. 2005 May;19(2):358-63.

De Bock K, Eijnde BO, Ramaekers M, Hespel P. Acute Rhodiola rosea intake can improve endurance exercise performance. Int J Sport Nutr Exerc Metab. 2004 Jun;14(3):298-307.

Earnest CP, Morss GM, Wyatt F, et al. Effects of a commercial herbal–based formula on exercise performance in cyclists. Med Sci Sports Exerc. 2004 Mar; 36(3):504-9.

Kim SH, Hyun SH, Choung SY. Antioxidative effects of Cinnamomi cassiae and Rhodiola rosea extracts in liver of diabetic mice. Biofactors. 2006;26(3):209-19.

Perfumi M, Mattioli L. Adaptogenic and central nervous system effects of single doses of 3% rosavin and 1% salidroside Rhodiola rosea L. extract in mice. Phytother Res. 2006 Oct 27.

Wing SL, Askew EW, Luetkemeier MJ, et al. Lack of effect of Rhodiola or oxygenated water supplementation on hypoxemia and oxidative stress. Wilderness Environ Med. 2003 Spring;14(1):9-16.

ф

Chapter
9

MISCELLANEOUS COMPOUNDS

This is a diverse group of compounds that don't fit neatly into any of the previous categories, but are nonetheless part of the bodybuilding pharmacopeia.

Each one is marketed to improve either body composition or performance through a variety of different mechanisms. How each one works—or is supposed to work—is covered in the following pages.

Miscellaneous Compounds Covered

❖ Caffeine

❖ Chocamine™

❖ Cissus Quadrangularis

❖ GH Supplements

❖ Glycerol

❖ MCTs

❖ Myostatin Inhibitors

❖ Saw Palmetto

CAFFEINE

What is it?

Caffeine is 1,3,7–trimethylxanthine, a naturally-occurring alkaloid in coffee, tea, and chocolate, as well as an additive in a number of commercial beverages, over-the-counter drugs, and supplements.

What is it supposed to do?

Caffeine is a stimulant that exerts a variety of physiological effects. Most of caffeine's major effects stem from its action as an adenosine receptor antagonist. When adenosine binds to receptors on the surface of neurons in the brain, neuronal activity slows down. By blocking those receptors, caffeine keeps neurons firing and facilitates the release of stimulatory neurotransmitters like adrenaline and noradrenaline, hence the "pick me up" sensation people get from a cup or two of coffee.

Caffeine exerts both positive and negative effects: it can increase thermogenesis, mitigate fatigue, enhance cognitive function, and improve athletic performance. It can also increase heart rate and blood pressure, cause insomnia, and—in sensitive individuals—induce gastrointestinal distress, anxiety, irritability, and other side effects.

One of the major downsides of caffeine is the fact the body becomes tolerant to chronic caffeine intake fairly quickly, and caffeine withdrawal can produce unpleasant symptoms such as headache, fatigue, and even nausea.

What does the research say for athletic performance?

Caffeine is one of the most heavily researched compounds in the world, and to give a full summary is beyond the scope of this review, which will focus on its effects on athletic performance and body composition.

Caffeine enhances exercise by delaying exercise-induced fatigue. In one cycling trial, for example, ingestion of 330 mg of caffeine 60 minutes before the test increased the time to exhaustion from an average of 75.5 minutes to 90.2 minutes. Another study showed that 250 mg x 2 doses of caffeine (one taken 60 minutes before exercise, the other consumed over the first 90 minutes of the exercise) showed a 7.4% increase in work production, and a 7.3% increase in VO2max. To take another example, runners consuming 4.45 mg/kg caffeine were able to increase their time to exhaustion by 7.5-10 minutes.

While caffeine does not appear to enhance strength performance, it has significant effects on mood and concentration. Subjects consuming caffeine are also able to perform more total work for the same level of perceived effort. This explains its popularity as a pre-workout supplement for strength athletes as well as endurance athletes.

One issue that has come up in recent research is the possible impact of caffeine on insulin resistance. A small study in 2002 demonstrated a 15% decrease in insulin sensitivity in lean, healthy volunteers who received a bolus of 3 mg/kg intravenous caffeine, followed by a steady infusion of 0.6 mg/kg for the duration of the experiment. Another study on lean, sedentary, nonsmoking men showed a 24% reduction in glucose uptake and a 35% decrease in carbohydrate storage.

Still another study showed that the reductions in insulin sensitivity persisted with caffeine ingestion, in spite of a three month aerobic exercise program, which might otherwise have improved insulin sensitivity.

There are several things to keep in mind: none of these studies have

1: been conducted on athletes, but relied on measurements of sedentary individuals for the most part. The one study that did look at exercise started with sedentary individuals and used "walking or light jogging on a treadmill for 60 min, five times per week at a moderate intensity (60% VO2max)" as the sole form of exercise.

So very fit people with potentially better insulin sensitivity have not been studied.

In support of this point, a study conducted by Thong et al., demonstrated that exercise did, in fact, improve post-caffeine insulin action. This study, however, used "...healthy, moderately active men" and used a one-leg knee extensor exercise protocol to look at insulin action in the exercised vs. non-exercised muscle.

All the studies looked at acute effects of caffeine ingestion, not chronic. Yet habitual caffeine intake induces tolerance to many of its effects. So none of the studies conducted so far tells us anything about chronic caffeine use, such as would be the case with using caffeine as a pre-workout stimulantor in an EC combo for fat loss.

2: The studies looked at the use of pure caffeine only, not consumption of caffeinated beverages, such as coffee. Furthermore, the doses were often quite high: 5 mg/kg, for example, is the equivalent to 500 mg for a 100 kg man. This is 2.5 times the amount in most caffeine–containing supplements (200 mg).

3: According to Thong, et al.,

"...the inhibitory effects of caffeine on glucose uptake occur only in the presence of high insulin levels" – so the impact of caffeine intake is likely to be mitigated by a diet with a low glycemic index as recommended in the book "Fat Loss Revealed."

So there is still plenty of room to debate the effects of chronic caffeine consumption on insulin sensitivity in athletes.

As alluded to above, the effects of drinking naturally caffeinated beverages like coffee makes it even more complicated. As it turns out, epidemiological studies have shown that coffee consumption may reduce the risk of developing diabetes as well as Metabolic Syndrome/Syndrome X! A recent review, "Coffee, Diabetes, and Weight Control" suggests that this may be due to the presence of non–caffeine components in coffee that counteract the effects of caffeine. Coffee contains chlorogenic acid and quinides which both enhance insulin sensitivity and glucose clearance in experimental animals. As the authors point out:

" It is not known whether tolerance develops to the effects of...other coffee compounds that have the ability to enhance insulin sensitivity. It may be that such tolerance does not develop, even though tolerance to caffeine's ability to depress insulin sensitivity does develop. If tolerance to the noncaffeine compounds does not develop, that could help explain the apparent contradiction between the long–term epidemiologic finding that coffee enhances glucose tolerance and the short–term finding that coffee impairs glucose tolerance. "

As is often the case, more research will be needed to clarify these points.

Another point of confusion concerning caffeine is the ongoing debate about whether or not caffeine interferes with creatine supplementation. The evidence that it does comes from two small studies performed by the same research group that concluded that caffeine completely negated the ergogenic effects of creatine use. These studies are generally not well–regarded and have not been replicated. In both, fairly large doses of caffeine were used: 5 mg/kg. Neither study actually looked at the effects on performance in a typical strength workout: the first used a series of extremely high repetition knee extensions; while the second looked at muscle relaxation times after electrical stimulation.

The funny thing is that many of the early studies looking at the positive effects of creatine supplementation on performance, used creatine dissolved in caffeine–containing beverages such as coffee and tea. So there may be a threshold for caffeine intake before it interferes with the effects of creatine—assuming, of course, that it has an effect at all.

For the record, people take caffeine and creatine all the time: lots of people are coffee drinkers, and/or take other caffeine–containing supplements (many NO supplements, diet supplements, and other pre-workout energizers like Red Bull) contain solid doses of caffeine). And quite a few take EC as well. I've yet to hear of anyone complain about any conflicts.

Thus, I'm inclined to not take the advice to avoid caffeine + creatine very seriously, pending of course, confirmation by some other group, using a study design that lends itself to drawing better real world conclusions.

What about real world athletic performance?

Caffeine is—to put it mildly—ubiquitous. It's in coffee, tea, and chocolate; it's in over-the-counter medications; it's included in the aforementioned energy drinks and supplements. I include a strong black cup of coffee in my pre-workout stack. Thousands of people use ephedrine and caffeine combos to lose excess fat. Most see caffeine as a benign, and often useful adjunct to their programs.

Will Brink's Recommendation

Caffeine is certainly useful as a workout energizer and ergogenic aid. As with any pharmacologically active compound, there are a few minuses to go along with the pluses.

Certainly some people are sensitive to it, and prefer to avoid it—although as far as this writer is concerned, there is no sunshine without coffee!

There are also some lingering questions about its role in reducing insulin sensitivity, but considering the large number of lean, healthy athletes who use it, my hunch is that future research will show that tolerance due to chronic use minimizes this problem—especially for people who are active and consume a healthy, low-GI diet. So caffeine still rates two thumbs up for athletes, at least in moderate amounts.

References

Cole KJ, Costill DL, Starling RD, et al. Effect of caffeine ingestion on perception of effort and subsequent work production. Int J Sport Nutr. 1996 Mar;6(1):14-23.

Costill DL, Dalsky GP, Fink WJ. Effects of caffeine ingestion on metabolism and exercise performance. Med Sci Sports. 1978 Fall;10(3):155-8.

Graham TE, Hibbert E, Sathasivam P. Metabolic and exercise endurance effects of coffee and caffeine ingestion. J Appl Physiol. 1998 Sep;85(3):883-9.

Greenberg JA, Boozer CN, Geliebter A. Coffee, diabetes, and weight control. Am J Clin Nutr. 2006 Oct;84(4):682-93.

Greer F, Hudson R, Ross R, Graham T. Caffeine ingestion decreases glucose disposal during a hyperinsulinemic–euglycemic clamp in sedentary humans. Diabetes. 2001 Oct;50(10):2349-54.

Haskell CF, Kennedy DO, Wesnes KA, Scholey AB. Cognitive and mood improvements of caffeine in habitual consumers and habitual non–consumers of caffeine. Psychopharmacology (Berl). 2005 Jun;179(4):813-25.

Hespel P, Op't Eijnde B, Van Leemputte M. Opposite actions of caffeine and creatine on muscle relaxation time in humans. J Appl Physiol. 2002 Feb; 92(2):513-8.

Ivy JL, Costill DL, Fink WJ, Lower RW. Influence of caffeine and carbohydrate feedings on endurance performance. Med Sci Sports. 1979 Spring;11(1):6-11.

Keijzers GB, De Galan BE, Tack CJ, Smits P. Caffeine can decrease insulin sensitivity in humans. Diabetes Care. 2002 Feb;25(2):364-9.

Lee S, Hudson R, Kilpatrick K, et al. Caffeine ingestion is associated with reductions in glucose uptake independent of obesity and type 2 diabetes before and after exercise training. Diabetes Care. 2005 Mar;28(3):566-72.

Thong FS, Derave W, Kiens B, et al. Caffeine–induced impairment of insulin action but not insulin signaling in human skeletal muscle is reduced by exercise. Diabetes. 2002 Mar;51(3):583-90.

Vandenberghe K, Gillis N, Van Leemputte M, et al. Caffeine counteracts the ergogenic action of muscle creatine loading. J Appl Physiol. 1996 Feb;80 (2):452-7.

ϙ

CISSUS QUADRANGULARIS

What is it?

Cissus quadrangularis is an edible plant found in India, Malaya, West Africa and Sri Lanka. In India, it's referred to as "bone setter," and is used to help heal fractures as well as treat ulcers, hemorrhoids, anorexia, indigestion, asthma, and wounds.

What is it supposed to do?

Cissus extracts are alleged to have analgesic and anabolic properties.

What does the research say for athletic performance?

Cissus extracts are used to treat a variety of ailments, so it's not surprising that the research is all over the map. For example, Cissus extracts have been found to have antimicrobial activity. A methanolic extract of Cissus quadrangularis was found to suppress the growth of both gram negative and gram positive bacteria in vitro: Bacillus subtilis, Pseudomonas aeruginosa, Salmonella typhi, Staphylococcus aureus, and Streptococcus pyogenes. In another study, Cissus quadrangularis extracts exhibited antibacterial activity against gram positive Bacillus, Staphylococcus and Streptococcus species.

Cissus extracts also possess antioxidant activity, and various compounds have been identified, including vitamin C, tannins, and flavonols. Additional potentially bioactive phytochemicals include sterols, saponins and triterpenoids.

Cissus extracts appear to have gastroprotective effects in animals with experimentally-induced ulcers. Rats given doses of 500 mg/kg showed an increase in mucosal protective factors, decreased inflammatory response and reduced tissue damage.

Cissus may also contribute to bone health. Cissus extracts given to ovariectomized rats at 500 and 750 mg/kg had anti–osteoporotic effects, while dogs with experimental fractures given 50 mg/kg Cissus extract (stems), healed more Cissus Quadrangularis quickly than the sham-treated group.

The one human study I found was concerned with weight loss, as well as improvement of risk factors for cardiovascular disease and metabolic syndrome. In this study, a commercial supplement (Cylaris^{TM}) containing Cissus quadrangularis was given to overweight or obese patients, with or without a 2100-2200 calorie diet. The obese subjects receiving the Cylaris^{TM} lost 6.6 kg (Cylaris^{TM} only) and 8.1 kg (Cylaris^{TM} and diet). Total cholesterol, as well as plasma triglycerides, C–reactive protein and fasting glucose also improved in the supplement groups. This study, however, did not look at the effects of Cissus alone.

The formula also contained green tea extract standardized for EGCG, which has also been found to have some effects on fat loss, so some of the weight loss and other measured differences may not be directly attributable to the Cissus.

Finally, Cissus extracts have been found to have analgesic and sedative effects in mice. Interparenteral doses of 50, 100, and 200 mg/kg produced 44%, 61% and 84% inhibition of chemically-induced writhing, respectively. Cissus administration also induced changes in motor coordination and exploratory behavior. A second study also demonstrated Cissus extracts reduced licking time and inhibited edema formation in experimentally-induced paw and ear inflammation in mice.

What about real world athletic performance?

Anecdotal reviews suggest that Cissus may have analgesic properties when taken orally. People who give Cissus high ratings claim that it reduces post-workout muscle and joint pain and accelerates healing of soft-tissue injuries. These statements are all subjective,and have not been backed up by any clinical evidence.

By all accounts, Cissus appears to be quite safe and free from any obvious adverse side effects. The recommended dose of extract is 500-1000 mg, and 3-6 g of dried plant powder.

Will Brink's Recommendation

While Cissus has a hallowed place in Ayurvedic medicine, the research backing it up as a supplement is tentative, at best. In this writer's opinion, the best evidence right now is anecdotal—so I can't recommend it at this time. It could be worth keeping an eye on, however, as more research is done.

References

Chidambara Murthy KN, Vanitha A, Mahadeva Swamy M, Ravishankar GA. Antioxidant and antimicrobial activity of Cissus quadrangularis L. J Med Food. 2003 Summer;6(2):99-105.

Deka DK, Lahon LC, Saikia J, Mukit A. Effect of Cissus quadrangularis in accelerating healing process of experimentally fractured radius–ulna of dog: a preliminary study. Indian J Pharmacol. 1994 26: 44-45.

Kashikar ND, George I. Antibacterial activity of Cissus quadrangularis Linn. Indian J Pharm Sci 2006;68:245-247.

Jainu M, Devi CS. Gastroprotective action of Cissus quadrangularis extract against NSAID induced gastric ulcer: role of proinflammatory cytokines and oxidative damage. Chem Biol Interact. 2006 Jul 10;161(3):262-70.

Jainu M, Devi CS. Effect of Cissus quadrangularis on gastric mucosal defensive factors in experimentally induced gastric ulcer—a comparative study with sucralfate. J Med Food. 2004 Fall;7(3):372-6.

Jainu M, Mohan KV, Devi CS. Protective effect of Cissus quadrangularis on neutrophil mediated tissue injury induced by aspirin in rats. J Ethnopharmacol. 2006 Apr 6;104(3):302-5.

Jainu M, Vijai Mohan K, Shyamala Devi CS. Gastroprotective effect of Cissus quadrangularis extract in rats with experimentally induced ulcer. Indian J Med Res. 2006 Jun;123(6):799-806.

Oben J, Kuate D, Agbor G, Momo C, Talla X. The use of a Cissus quadrangularis formulation in the management of weight loss and metabolic syndrome. Lipids Health Dis. 2006 Sep 2;5:24.

Panthong A, Supraditaporn W, Kanjanapothi D, Taesotikul T et al. Analgesic, anti-inflammatory and venotonic effects of Cissus quadrangularis Linn. J Ethnopharmacol. 2007 Mar 21;110(2):264-70.

Shirwaikar A, Khan S, Malini S. Antiosteoporotic effect of ethanol extract of Cissus quadrangularis Linn. on ovariectomized rat. J Ethnopharmacol. 2003 Dec;89(2–3):245-50.

Viswanatha Swamy AHM, Thippeswamy AHM, Manjula DV, Mahendra Kumar CB. Some Neuropharmacological Effects of the Methanolic Root Extract of Cissus Quadrangularis in Mice. Afr J Biomed Res. 2006 Vol. 9:69-75.

ॐ

CHOCAMINE™

What is it?

Chocamine™ is a propietary cocoa extract produced by RFI Ingredients, a manufacturer of botanicals and nutraceuticals. Chocamine™ is—in RFI's words—

"...a proprietary, patent pending cocoa extract that has the taste, smell and proven health benefits of chocolate without the sugar, fat and dairy of chocolate candy."

What is it supposed to do?

Chocamine™—like cocoa—contains a variety of bioactive compounds, some of which are known to have different effects on mood, performance and fat oxidation. Thus, Chocamine™ is most often found in workout boosters and/or fat loss supplements.

What does the research say for athletic performance?

There is no research specifically on Chocamine™. There is, however, plenty of research on cocoa, and—as a cocoa extract—presumably what is true for cocoa is also true for Chocamine™, although this depends on the methods of producing the extract. Cocoa compounds may be lost, or present in proportions somewhat different in the extract vs. the starting material.

Cocoa contains a number of biologically active compounds, such as:

– methylxanthines (caffeine, theobromine, theophylline)

– biogenic amines (phenylethylamine, tyramine)

– amino acids

– essential minerals (magnesium, copper)

– polyphenols (esp. flavan–3–ols, procyanidins)

Of these classes of compounds, cocoa polyphenols have received the most attention, due to their role as antioxidants, and potential modulators of cardiovascular risk. Cocoa polyphenols have been found to improve vasodilation and reduce blood pressure, inhibit platelet activity and decrease inflammation.

Cocoa is also a source of caffeine, as well as other methylxanthines which have effects on mood, energy and cognition. Biogenic amines are a diverse group of compounds, which include human neurotransmitters such as dopamine, serotonin, and epinephrine. The biogenic amines present in cocoa include tyramine, which can cause vasoconstriction and increased blood pressure, and phenylethylamine, which has (debatable) psychological effects. Tyramine is an ingredient in several OTC diet supplements, due to it's (experimental) ability to improve glucose disposal and stimulate/postentiate the release of norepinephrine.

Thus, Chocamine™ could work on several different levels: as a source of antioxidants, as a stimulant, and—possibly—for fat loss, but this is somewhat speculative, since only the amounts of a few compounds are known.

Chocamine™ contains approximately 8% caffeine, 12% theobromine, and ~3.5% polyphenols (in other words, 80 mg, 120 mg, and 35 mg per gram, respectively).

What about real world athletic performance?

Chocamine™ certainly appears to have stimulant effects. Users report that it gives a smoother "buzz" than caffeine alone, although it does appear to induce tolerance with constant use.

Will Brink's Recommendation

Chocamine™'s main value appears to be as a workout booster, and it gets a thumbs up for this purpose. It seems to work best when taken on an empty stomach. A dose of 500 mg-2 grams is fairly typical. It's often found in bulk powder form, and is not particularly expensive, although it is extremely bitter-tasting and is better to use capped.

References

Burchett SA, Hicks TP. The mysterious trace amines: protean neuromodulators of synaptic transmission in mammalian brain. Prog Neurobiol. 2006 Aug;79(5–6):223-46.

Engler MB, Engler MM. The emerging role of flavonoid–rich cocoa and chocolate in cardiovascular health and disease. Nutr Rev. 2006 Mar;64(3):109-18.

Steinberg FM, Bearden MM, Keen CL. Cocoa and chocolate flavonoids: implications for cardiovascular health. J Am Diet Assoc. 2003 Feb;103(2):215-23.

Visentin V, Bour S, Boucher J, Prevot D, et. al. Glucose handling in streptozotocin–induced diabetic rats is improved by tyramine but not by the amine oxidase inhibitor semicarbazide. Eur J Pharmacol. 2005 Oct 17;522(1-3):139-46.

♄

CLA (CONJUGATED LINOLEIC ACID)

What is it?

CLA (Conjugated Linoleic Acid) is found predominantly in dairy products and it appears to be a fatty acid with some unique effects on the metabolism of animals and (hopefully) people. CLA is not a single substance: rather, it's a series of isomers of linoleic acid with conjugated bonds ("conjugated" = two double bonds separated by a single bond). The CLA found in milk/meat is predominantly the cis–9, trans–11 isomer (also known as "rumenic acid"). Commercial supplements, on the other hand, are a mixture of isomers, dominated by the cis–9, trans–11 and trans–10, cis–12 isomers.

What is it supposed to do?

As readers of this book may recall, we have looked at the topic of lipids/fats in sports nutrition, fat loss, etc. and come to the conclusion that not all fats are "bad" and some may help performance, body fat levels and strength. ConjugatedLinoleic Acid (CLA) may very well be just such a fat.

What does the research say for athletic performance?

Several in vitro (test tube) and animal studies have shown it has powerful antioxidant properties as well as impressive anti-cancer properties. It has been shown to modulate insulin–like growth factor binding proteins (IGFBP's) in mice and may also improve insulin sensitivity. It has been shown to suppress the growth of certain lines of human breast cancer as well as several other cancers. Animals subjected to various cancer causing chemicals and fed CLA appear to fare much better than those not getting CLA. Some studies with CLA also point to this lipid as a possible immune enhancer.

"This is all very interesting and wonderful, but I want to know what it can do for athletes?" the reader is thinking. Well, since this is a sports supplement oriented book we will stick to that angle.

Perhaps more relevant and interesting to athletes, CLA has been found to be the best thing for building muscle and losing fat in mice and rats since they slipped anabolic steroids in their mouse food! A substantial number of studies has confirmed that animals (the aforementioned squeaky things with red eyes) add lean body mass in the form of muscle and lose body fat when fed CLA, making CLA a true anabolic agent in rodents.

"Ok," we are all thinking, "Lots of things work on mice and rats but this doesn't seem to do a thing for us higher animals lifting weights." That is true. And like many supplements, the human data are lacking; yet growing steadily. The good news is we have a few notable human studies. The bad news is they continue to be conflicting in their findings.

Pertaining to building muscle, research was presented at a large conference in Lahti, Finland recently by a Dr. Lowery. The study fed 24 novice bodybuilders 12 grams of a product containing 7.2 grams of CLA or placebo (vegetable oil) while completing a 6 week program of bodybuilding exercises. The study found the group getting CLA had an increase in strength and arm girth (their arms got larger) but did not add body fat leaving the researchers to conclude,

"apparently, CLA acts as a mild anabolic agent in novice male bodybuilders."

One recent study found that CLA supplementation at 3-4 grams per day caused an almost one inch reduction in waist size and a loss of body fat of 2-4 lb in overweight subjects over a 12 week period. Additonal studies have also shown positive effects. One long term study on 134 overweight men and women showed statistically significant fat loss over the first 6 months of a 24 month study. The study also demonstrated that fat-free mass was preserved, and that the dose of CLA supplied (3.4 g/day) was safe and had no long term adverse effects. Another 6 month study on 40 overweight subjects receiving 3.2 g/day CLA had similar results. A study on twenty normal weight, exercising volunteers also showed statistically significant fat loss using 1.8 g/day CLA for 12 weeks.

But, a pilot study using weight lifters found no differences in body weight, fat, or muscle mass over a 30 day period. Another small study with ten subjects, receiving 3-4 grams of CLA versus 10 subjects getting a placebo for three months, found similar results. A third study of 17 healthy women getting 3 grams of CLA versus placebo (sunflower oil) for 64 days, found no statistically significant differences between the two groups.

To complicate the picture, other research has suggested that CLA can a) enhance the formation of inflammatory cytokines; b) have unfavorable effects on blood lipids; and c) increase insulin resistance. These effects appear to be isomer-specific. For example, one study showed that the trans–10, cis–12 isomer increased insulin resistance by 19% and reduced HDL cholesterol in men with abdominal obesity.

Studies on supplementation with the mixed isomers, however, do not appear to produce such detrimental changes. One recent study on 41 healthy overweight adults published in the International Journal of Obesity concluded that after 6 months of supplementation:

" CLA does not affect glucose metabolism or insulin sensitivity in a population of overweight or obese volunteers."

This was echoed by the researchers in the 24 month safety study mentioned earlier who concluded:

" CLA was well tolerated and the observed changes in the safety variables were all within the normal range, suggesting that CLA supplementation in healthy, overweight subjects for 24 mo is safe."

Yet another study on healthy, overweight volunteers using 6 g of CLA in the form of a commercial supplement (Clarinol) for 12 months also concluded that there were no adverse effects on blood glucose, lipids, or insulin levels.

What about real world athletic performance?

Feedback from users has been mixed, although there are people who feel they've gotten positive results from using CLA. Although many of the human studies have used ~3 g a day, the most positive comments have come from those using 6-7 g/day.

Will Brink's Recommendation

Although some of the findings with CLA in people have been exciting and interesting, there continues to be too many conflicting studies. Though it may turn out to be a worthwhile supplement for athletes, far more human research is needed for definitive conclusions, but CLA is a supplement to keep an eye on.

For increasing muscle mass or improving performance, it gets a thumbs down until more human research is done. As a fat loss agent, it may be worth a try but again, research is conflicting at best. I'd say fish oils are a better bang for that use. At this point, even though I am giving it a thumbs down for building muscle, I consider it one of those "might be worth a try" supplements.

References

Banni S, Angioni E, Casu V, et al. Decrease in linoleic acid metabolites as a potential mechanism in cancer risk reduction by conjugated linoleic acid. Carcinogenesis. 1999 Jun;20(6):1019-24.

Basu S, Riserus U, Turpeinen A, Vessby B. Conjugated linoleic acid induces lipid peroxidation in men with abdominal obesity. Clin Sci (Lond). 2000 Dec;99(6):511-6.

Li Y, Seifert MF, Ney DM, et al. Dietary conjugated linoleic acids alter serum IGF–I and IGF binding protein concentrations and reduce bone formation in rats fed (n–6) or (n–3) fatty acids. J Bone Miner Res. 1999 Jul;14(7):1153-62.

Lowery LM, Appicelli PA, Lemon PW. Conjugated Linoleic Acid Enhances Muscle Size and strength Gains in Novice Bodybuilders. 1998. Med. Sci. Sports Excercise. 30(5).

Gaullier JM, Halse J, Hoye K, et al. Supplementation with conjugated linoleic acid for 24 months is well tolerated by and reduces body fat mass in healthy, overweight humans. J Nutr. 2005 Apr;135(4):778-84.

Park Y, Storkson JM, Albright KJ, et al. Evidence that the trans–10,cis–12 isomer of conjugated linoleic acid induces body composition changes in mice. Lipids. 1999 Mar;34(3):235-41.

Syvertsen C, Halse J, Hoivik HO, et al. The effect of 6 months supplementation with conjugated linoleic acid on insulin resistance in overweight and obese. Int J Obes (Lond). 2006 Oct 10.

Thom E, Wadstein J, Gudmundsen O. Conjugated linoleic acid reduces body fat in healthy exercising humans. J Int Med Res. 2001 Sep–Oct;29(5):392-6.

Watras AC, Buchholz AC, Close RN, et al. The role of conjugated linoleic acid in reducing body fat and preventing holiday weight gain. Int J Obes (Lond). 2006 Aug 22.

Whigham LD, O'Shea M, Mohede IC, et al. Safety profile of conjugated linoleic acid in a 12–month trial in obese humans. Food Chem Toxicol. 2004 Oct;42(10):1701-9.

Zambell KL, Keim NL, Van Loan MD, et al. Conjugated linoleic acid supplementation in humans: effects on body composition and energy expenditure. Lipids. 2000 Jul;35(7):777-82.

GH SUPPLEMENTS

What are they?

There is a long list of supplements being sold claiming to be either Human Growth Hormone (HGH or GH), or to cause the release of GH. The number of nutrients claiming to be able to increase HGH levels is long.

The major products in this category currently being, marketed can be broken down into three major categories:

- Homeopathic GH claiming to contain actual HGH
- Growth hormone promoting nutrients (certain amino acids, vitamins,etc.)
- Secretagogues, short peptides that supposedly, cause a release of GH.

What are they supposed to do?

Increase the production of growth hormone, which will help increase muscle mass and or decrease body fat levels.

What does the research say for athletic performance?

The role of GH in the human body is extensive and rather complicated with many effects still being elucidated. GH is known to play an essential role in the regulation of body fat levels, immunity, muscle mass, wound healing, bone mass, and literally thousands of other functions both known and yet unknown. Real human GH is a peptide 191 amino acids long with a molecular weight of approximately 20,000.

It is produced by the anterior pituitary gland, located at the base of the brain. The bulk of the effect accomplished by GH is performed by a related hormone (Insulin–like Growth Factor–1 or IGF–1), which is released predominantly by the liver and, to some extent, by other tissues in response to GH levels. However, some recent data suggest GH has effects separate from that of its relation to IGF–1.

It is well established that GH levels steadily decline as we age and is partially responsible for the steady loss of muscle mass, loss of skin elasticity, immune dysfunction, and many other physical changes that take place in the aging human body. Explaining in detail the many roles GH plays in the human body is beyond the scope of this book.

Research with GH has been both interesting and conflicting. However, the bulk of research with actual injections of GH is compelling. In populations that have reduced GH levels—such as the elderly—injections of GH have been shown to: increase skin thickness and elasticity, improve healing time and reduce infection rates after surgery, decrease body fat, increase muscle mass, increase bone density, improve cholesterol levels (by decreasing LDL cholesterol and increasing HDL cholesterol), and improve exercise capacity. GH–releasing nutrients claim to release GH and thus have the positive effects associated with GH.

The number of nutrients found to possibly cause a release of GH are many, and include the amino acids arginine, leucine, ornithine, and glutamine; vitamins such as niacin, choline and pantothenic acid, and non–vitamin nutrients such as melatonin, as well as many others. Although there is a good deal of data showing many of these nutrients can cause a release of GH to some degree, not one study has demonstrated the same effects in humans or animals, as is seen with actual injections of GH as outlined above.

Other products claim to contain actual GH in extremely minute quantities, which is the nature of homeopathic products, which is they dilute a compound (in this case GH) down to virtually undetectable levels and claim it still has biological effects. Regarding GH, this idea is full of problems. For one, the amounts found in these products are of no biological significance, and even if directly injected at those levels, would have no effects on muscle mass or body fat levels. Another major issue is the fact that GH is a very delicate molecule and will not survive the digestive process as the 191 amino acid length of GH will be chopped up by digestive enzymes. There is no sold data showing any of these products effect muscle mass or body fat. So a thumbs down for homeopathic GH supps.

A secretagogue is a generally made up of short peptides, 6-11 amino acids long, that may survive the digestive process and are orally absorbable. This has been an intensive area of research for pharmaceutical companies looking for a better way to increase GH levels instead of injections.

Some studies have shown these pharmaceutical compounds can stimulate the production of significant amounts of GH. For example, one secretagogue made by the huge pharmaceutical company Merck, is called NK677. Research looking at NK677 found it increased the GH pulse during GH production and increased the frequency of the GH pulse.

Did this natural "pulse" of GH have an improved anabolic response over big single injections as studied in the previous research mentioned above? The answer appeared to be no, as there were no changes in muscle mass, strength or body fat in young weight lifters or older people who were given NK677. To date, there is no data showing any of the "natural" secretagogues being sold on the supplement market alter body fat, muscle mass, or performance, much less the real pharmaceutical versions that are still being researched.

The problems with this category of supplements are many. For example, the age and GH status of the person appear to have a great deal to do with any released GH, and many factors will dictate how much if any, GH does get released. I have not listed doses for the above nutrients because they vary so greatly, nutrient to nutrient. Some data also suggest that other counter regulatory hormones such as the catabolic (muscle wasting) hormone cortisol may go up in response to such products.

None of the GH releasing products listed above have ever been shown to keep GH levels sustained and/or reach high enough levers—as injections of real GH have achieved—which appears necessary to see any real effects in body fat levels or muscle mass.

Also, in younger individuals with normal GH levels, even GH injections seem to be of little to no benefit. However, when combined with other hormones, such as anabolic steroids, many people feel regular GH injections (not supplements!) do have a synergism together that leads to greater increases in LBM and reductions in body fat than would be seen by either used alone. In the off season, some high level bodybuilders have used the stack known as "the big three" which refers to the use of testosterone, GH, and insulin combined. No doubt, this is a very potent combination of hormones. However, we have no real data to go on with this 'magic' combo in healthy athletes.

The benefits of GH injections may be of real use to older populations that suffer from low GH levels, and many bodybuilders feel it assists in losing body fat and retaining LBM pre-contest. The truth is, GH levels go up and down all the time and can be altered by all sorts of things, from exercise, to standing in the cold, to hitting yourself on the head with a hammer…

Even if the current "GH releasing" products on the market do have some effects on GH (and I am not convinced they do), there is no reason to believe at this time they will effect muscle mass or body fat.

Sellers of such products make them look like the best thing since sliced bread by listing all the known effects of GH in the human body, then pretending their products have been proven to mimic those effects. The problem is they have not been shown to do this and probably never will. Even much of the research using injections of real GH is often conflicting.

For example, one study looked at both young and old people given fairly large doses of GH and put on a weight lifting program. Both groups were given 40 mcg per kg of GH daily, which is a good sized dose. This research found that GH didn't increase protein synthesis or decrease protein breakdown (anti catabolism) in the young guys lifting weights, even though their IGF–1 levels tripled. Also, there were no changes in strength between the GH group and the placebo group.

In the older group, the guys getting the GH did gain more fat free mass (FFM) than the placebo group. However, the additional FFM turned out to be almost all water and not actual protein accumulation in the group getting the GH. Both groups showed similar strength increases.

So, in total, the amount of actual muscle gained by the older group getting GH was "nada" and it didn't do anything for their strength either.

Their conclusion was that large doses of GH combined with weight training has no additive effects over that of just weight training and IGF–1 levels went up without anabolic effect.

They did however feel that small multiple doses of GH would work better than one large whopping dose as this study used.

What about real world athletic performance?

There are a great many products on the market, and most of these are a mixture of various nutrients known to cause transient spikes in GH levels. While a few experience very modest effects, it's safe to say that no one has ever lost a significant amount of fat, nor gained a significant amount of muscle by using them. This goes double for the various oral or "sublingual" GH preparations sold in health food stores or on the internet.

As alluded to above about supplements that claim to raise GH, it's one thing to raise the level of some hormone, but a totally different thing to show that a raise in that hormone is leading to more muscle mass or less body fat. That is, who cares if the product raises some hormone, if in the end, it has no effect on muscle mass or body fat?!

Will Brink's Recommendation

This is not to say that GH does not play an important role in the body as a regulator of muscle growth and fat loss, but it is very clear that it is far more complicated than simply raising this hormone by injection or supplements. Another important thing to know: chronically high GH levels are not by default a good thing and can come with side effects over time, such as insulin resistance, various neuropathies, and other problems. Many bodybuilders I know personally have had to get their wrists operated on to relieve the pain of carpal tunnel syndrome they experienced from high dose injection of GH. It's not as uncommon as you may think in the higher ranks of bodybuilding, in fact, and is not something that gets coverage in the mags.

For older individuals who have confirmed low GH levels, GH therapy by injections given by a medical doctor might be worth pursuing. As for safety, the GH releasing supplements appear safe enough. At this time, I give GH supplements a thumbs down.

☧

GLYCEROL

What is it?

Glycerol (1,2,3–propanetriol) is an integral component of the triglyceride molecule. As most people who have taken a basic nutrition or biology course will tell you, glycerol forms the backbone of the triglyceride molecule, which is one of several ways the body transfers fat around in the body. If you break up a triglyceride, you will get three free fatty acids and glycerol (hence the reason It's called the backbone of a triglyceride).

Glycerol is defined as a naturally occurring trivalent alcohol. Similar to carbohydrates, glycerol oxidation yields 4.32 kcals per gram. So even though the number of calories in carbohydrates and glycerol are the same, structurally, they aren't the same.

What is it supposed to do?

Glycerol is a nutrient that has gotten some attention in the bodybuilding magazines as a supposed "plasma expander" and is hocked as having some ability to increase the fullness of muscles. It's also added to MRP bars for its mild sweet taste and gives the bar good texture similar to fat. Glycerol is used in the food industry to improve moisture, palatability and as a sweetener.

What does the research say for athletic performance?

Over the past few years, there has been a great deal of confusion over exactly what glycerol is and what it is not. It's neither a carb, nor a fat, although it can be utilized for energy.

When the body is starved of both calories and carbohydrates, under the right conditions, it will convert certain non-carbohydrate substrates to glucose, such as glycerol, certain amino acids, etc. This is not major source of carbohydrates (glucose) under normal conditions. Under normal conditions, i.e. when a person is eating normally (not starving), you can consume enough glycerol to fill an elephant, but there are not large changes in blood glucose and insulin.

For example, in one study, six healthy, non-obese men ingested either glucose, glycerol or a placebo during exercise to exhaustion on a cycle ergometer (73 percent of VO2max). The ingestion of glucose (1 gram per kg body weight, equal to 70 grams for a 150 lb person) 45 minutes prior to exercise produced a 50 percent increase in plasma glucose, as well as a three-fold increase in plasma insulin at zero minutes of exercise. On the other hand, glycerol consumption (1 gram per kg body weight) 45 minutes prior to exercise produced a 340-fold increase in plasma glycerol; but resting levels of plasma glucose and insulin did not change.

Is there any use to glycerol in the diet? Possibly. Dr. Jose Antonio suggests that substituting glycerol for high-glycemic carbohydrates could minimize the plethora of health problems associated with eating cookies and cakes and other very high GI foods.

Is glycerol a legitimate ergogenic aid? Since glycerol enables one to retain more fluid, some scientists theorize that taking exogenous glycerol might help performance. This is based on the fact that if one is well hydrated, one will be able to train harder and longer, particularly in hot environments. Some studies have found mild improvements in endurance athletes given glycerol but studies have been mixed with some finding no effect. As with all science, there isn't a unanimous consensus on glycerol's effects. Some sports nutrition companies sell glycerol to bodybuilders as a "plasma expander" since glycerol can pull fluids into the vascular system temporarily and may enhance the pump you feel in the gym, or when stepping on stage.

What about real world athletic performance?

So far the feedback on such a strategy is mixed, with many athletes reporting a crushing headache after ingesting large amounts of glycerol. Glycerol monostearate—a monoglyceride which is the latest form of supplemental glycerol—may work better for this purpose. Several supplements on the market use glycerol monostearate. The feedback has been mixed with regard to the pump, but there appear to be fewer complaints of side effects.

Will Brink's Recommendation

Glycerol does not appear to have any major effects on hydration or endurance. As far as strength training goes, it's only major use appears to be cosmetic: looking pumped may be good for one's ego, but it does little to add to real mass or strength. As an additive to low carb protein bars and other products, I give it a thumbs up, but as a workout supplement, I give it a thumbs down.

References

Gleeson M, Maughan RJ, Greenhaff PL. Comparison of the effects of pre-exercise feeding of glucose, glycerol and placebo on endurance and fuel homeostasis in man. Eur J Appl Physiol Occup Physiol. 1986;55(6):645-53.

Kavouras SA, Armstrong LE, Maresh CM, et al. Rehydration with glycerol: endocrine, cardiovascular, and thermoregulatory responses during exercise in the heat. J Appl Physiol. 2006 Feb;100(2):442-50.

Miller JM, Coyle EF, Sherman WM, et al. Effect of glycerol feeding on endurance and metabolism during prolonged exercise in man. Med Sci Sports Exerc. 1983;15(3):237-42.

Montner P, Stark DM, Riedesel ML, et al. Pre-exercise glycerol hydration improves cycling endurance time. Int J Sports Med. 1996 Jan;17(1):27-33.

Murray R, Eddy DE, Paul GL, et al. Physiological responses to glycerol ingestion during exercise. J Appl Physiol. 1991 Jul;71(1):144-9.

Wagner DR. Hyperhydrating with glycerol: implications for athletic performance. J Am Diet Assoc. 1999 Feb;99(2):207-12.

⚱

MEDIUM CHAIN TRIGLYCERIDES (MCTs)

What is it?

MCTs are technically saturated fats with 8–10 carbons, making them "medium" length fatty acids (the long chain fatty acids that make up food fats/oils typically have 16, 18, or more, carbons). MCT's can be produced by fractionating other oils, such as coconut oil.

What is it supposed to do?

MCTs are supposed to increase thermogenesis and help burn body fat. They are also promoted as a source of surplus calories for bulking that are less likely to be stored as body fat.

What does the research say for athletic performance?

What if there were a fat you could eat that was not stored as body fat and would just be burned off as heat? Would this be the nirvana of fat loss supplements and free energy source for athletes?

Well the proponents of Medium Chain Triglycerides (MCTs) would certainly like us to believe that MCTs are the answer to athletes' and dieters' dreams. Is it true?

Sort of.

Because of their shorter length, MCTs are processed differently in the body and can bypass many steps that long chain fatty acids must go through to be used as energy and stored as body fat. For example, long chain fatty acids must be transported to the mitochondria (the "power house" of cells) via something called the carnitine shuttle system.

This system is one of several limiting steps in the amount and rate of fat that can be "burned" or oxidized for energy at any one time. MCTs, on the other hand, can bypass this shuttle system and can enter the mitochondria directly to be used as energy. This is one of several reasons MCTs are considered less likely to be stored as body fat than long chain fatty acids.

Some studies in both people and animals suggests MCTs increase the thermic effect of food and increase daily energy expenditure (EE); which means the energy is lost as heat rather than stored as body fat. However, the few studies that have looked directly at the use of MCT's for weight loss in humans have been disappointing.

More often than not, studies that looked at MCT's for weight loss in people have found minimal effects. The reason is not totally clear, but it may because some of the positive effects of MCT's are offset by several negative effects on metabolism. For example, there may be an increased production of triglycerides and an increased release of the fat storage hormone insulin from ingesting MCT oils. There is some limited evidence that they may be of some value as replacements for LCTs in very low carbohydrate diets, but that's all.

Studies on the uses of MCTs to enhance athletic performance have been equally disappointing. MCTs don't spare the use of glycogen during endurance exercise, and don't improve performance. MCT consumption even impaired sprint performance in one study.

There are other possible drawbacks to MCTs. For example, MCTs don't contain fat soluble vitamins such as vitamin E, D, and K, nor do they contain any essential fatty acids (EFAs). MCTs do appear to have some genuine medical uses where digestion of fats and various liver problems exist, as well as having possible anti-catabolic (muscle sparing) effects in hospitalized patients.

What about real world athletic performance?

Though MCTs may not be the nirvana of fat loss products and energy enhancers some people make it out to be, there may still be a place for this product in the athletes arsenal of supplements and some experimentation is recommended. Some athletes find MCTs to be useful within the context of a keto diet, or as a source of extra, easily metabolized calories.

Will Brink's Recommendation

People who push MCTs as some sort of muscle building, anabolic fat are feeding people a load of you know what. For building muscle and or improving strength and performance, MCTs get a thumbs down at this time. Bang for the buck, flax oil and fish oils are better money spent, and the data much more consistent that they can positively impact body composition. Getting small amounts of MCT's from sources such as coconut oil and others may be useful to an overall nutrition program, but claims are exaggerated at best.

References

Bach AC, Ingenbleek Y, Frey A. The usefulness of dietary medium–chain triglycerides in body weight control: fact or fancy? J Lipid Res. 1996 Apr;37(4):708-26.

Goedecke JH, Clark VR, Noakes TD, Lambert EV. The effects of medium–chain triacylglycerol and carbohydrate ingestion on ultra–endurance exercise performance. Int J Sport Nutr Exerc Metab. 2005 Feb;15(1):15-27.

Krotkiewski M. Value of VLCD supplementation with medium chain triglycerides. Int J Obes Relat Metab Disord. 2001 Sep;25(9):1393-400.

Misell LM, Lagomarcino ND, Schuster V, Kern M. Chronic medium–chain triacylglycerol consumption and endurance performance in trained runners. J Sports Med Phys Fitness. 2001 Jun;41(2):210-5.

Papamandjaris AA, MacDougall DE, Jones PJ. Medium chain fatty acid metabolism and energy expenditure: obesity treatment implications. Life Sci. 1998; 62(14):1203-15.

St–Onge MP, Jones PJ. Greater rise in fat oxidation with medium–chain triglyceride consumption relative to long–chain triglyceride is associated with lower initial body weight and greater loss of subcutaneous adipose tissue. Int J Obes Relat Metab Disord. 2003 Dec;27(12):1565-71.

☧

MYOSTATIN INHIBITORS

What is it?

The current supplements claiming to be "myostatin inhibitors" are based on a seaweed extract that (supposedly) was found to bind to myostatin in a test tube (in vitro). I don't think it takes a science degree to see that this idea is based on flimsy science at best, and wishful thinking and good marketing at worst.

What is it supposed to do?

Myostatin is a member of a superfamily of related compounds known as "transforming growth factors beta." They are intimately related to tissue growth and differentiation, as well as many other functions. What scientists discovered was by knocking out the gene that codes for myostatin (the famed "myostatin gene"), animals would grow up hugely muscular. One needs only to see pictures of that ridiculously muscular mouse in the supplement ads to know what I mean. So the idea behind these supplements is that blocking myostatin will enable muscle growth.

What does the research say for athletic performance?

Scientists have been looking at these growth factors since they may have applications to grow livestock with greater amounts of meat and less fat, or combating wasting syndromes in humans, such as AIDS, cancer, and muscular dystrophy.

For example, high levels of myostatin have been associated with muscle wasting in HIV–infected men compared to healthy normal men. However, this simple association does not in anyway prove myostatin directly contributes to muscle wasting, per se. It may simply be an intermediate indicator vs. a direct cause. Myostatin may be one way the body regulates lean tissue growth (muscle) and appears to be a direct inhibitor of skeletal muscle growth, at least in prenatal and perhaps growing animals, but its effects in adult animals—much less adult humans—is very poorly understood at this time. Further research is needed to determine whether myostatin even plays a role in muscle growth after birth and in adults.

Relating to bodybuilders and other athletes, one theory is that the reason some people put on muscle so much easier than others is that they have a genetic propensity for making less myostatin due to a mutation in the gene. Conversely, the reason some people find it almost impossible to add muscle might be that they are genetically set up to have high levels of myostatin and, therefore, their efforts in the gym are being blocked. That overly simple theory is all well and fine, but data has been contradictory at best.

One group of researchers compared different groups of people to their level of muscularity and race and found that mutations in the human myostatin gene had little impact on responses in muscle mass to strength training. The fact is, muscle regeneration of injured skeletal muscle tissue, that is exactly how muscle heals itself in response to say weight training, is an extremely complex system that is not well understood.

To say that scientists, much less supplement companies, don't fully understand the roles of myostatin in exercise-induced muscle hypertrophy or regeneration following exercise, is putting it mildly. Myostatin probably plays an essential role as a regulator of LBM in adult humans as recent data suggests, but what role and how it works, is still to be elucidated.

Ok, bottom line here is, scientists know very little about how or if myostatin plays a direct role in muscle tissue of adult healthy human athletes. It's also absolutely essential that people understand that all such systems in the human body are under the control of an immensely complicated system of checks and balances, multi–layered feedback pathways, some of which are known, many of which are not.

There is a reason the body regulates anabolic and catabolic processes so tightly, and altering that very delicate balance can have unforeseen long–term effects. It's interesting to note that one pharmaceutical company has applied for a patent (United States Patent #6,369,201) that is an antibody to myostatin, and would reduce myostatin levels. There is no doubt that the research looking into the effects of myostatin on LBM of healthy and sick people is an interesting and worthwhile pursuit by researchers, but as a supplement to spend money on, it is premature to say the least.

The current crop of supplements contain sulfated polysaccharides from brown seaweed (Cystoseira canariensis). Why brown seaweed? This is because polysaccharides isolated from brown seaweed were found to bind to serum myostatin in an in vitro (test tube) experiment. Needless to state, what happens in a test tube can be quite different from what happens when a compound is consumed and digested.

This was demonstrated rather conclusively by a 2004 study that fed 1200 mg/day of a commercial myostatin inhibitor to untrained males participating in a 12 week resistance training program. The study concluded:

"Twelve wk of heavy resistance training and 1200 mg/d of Cystoseira canariensis supplementation appears ineffective at inhibiting serum myostatin and increasing muscle strength and mass or decreasing fat mass."

What about real world athletic performance?

Do you even need to ask? Commercial supplements based on Cystoseira canariensis (a.k.a. brown seaweed) are quietly fading into oblivion.

Will Brink's Recommendation

There has been mention in the mags of an in vivo study with people, with results on LBM that seemed far too good to be true (what else is new!). Until such a study is published in a peer reviewed Western/legit journal (most scientists have little faith in Eastern Bloc research or journals as they often lack the same stringent quality control western research/journals are subjected to) by an independent source not associated with the company making these supplements, I see no reason for people to spend their hard earned money on such a product at this time.

Perhaps companies selling these supplements will fund some studies in adult humans showing they have some effects on muscle mass, strength, or performance, but until then, they get a big thumbs down from me at this time.

References

Gonzalez–Cadavid NF, Taylor WE, Yarasheski K, et al. Organization of the human myostatin gene and expression in healthy men and HIV–infected men with muscle wasting. Proc Natl Acad Sci U S A. 1998 Dec 8;95(25):14938-43.

McPherron AC, Lee SJ. Double muscling in cattle due to mutations in the myostatin gene. Proc Natl Acad Sci U S A. 1997 Nov 11;94(23):12457-61.

Ramazanov Z, Jimenez del Rio M, Ziegenfuss T. R. Sulfated polysaccharides of brown seaweed Cystoseira canariensis bind to serum myostatin protein.Acta Physiol Pharmacol Bulg. 2003;27(2–3):101-6.

Sakuma K, Watanabe K, Sano M, et al. Differential adaptation of growth and differentiation factor 8/myostatin, fibroblast growth factor 6 and leukemia inhibitory factor in overloaded, regenerating and denervated rat muscles. Biochim Biophys Acta. 2000 Jun 2;1497(1):77-88.

Lee SJ, McPherron AC. Regulation of myostatin activity and muscle growth. Proc Natl Acad Sci U S A. 2001 Jul 31;98(16):9306–11. Epub 2001 Jul 17. Sharma M, Langley B, Bass J, Kambadur R. Myostatin in muscle growth and repair. Exerc Sport Sci Rev. 2001 Oct;29(4):155-8.

Willoughby DS. Effects of an alleged myostatin–binding supplement and heavy resistance training on serum myostatin, muscle strength and mass, and body composition. Int J Sport Nutr Exerc Metab. 2004 Aug;14(4):461-72.

Yamanouchi K, Soeta C, Naito K, Tojo H. Expression of myostatin gene in regenerating skeletal muscle of the rat and its localization. Biochem Biophys Res Commun. 2000 Apr 13;270(2):510-6.

Ϙ

SAW PALMETTO

What is it?

Saw palmetto (SP) is from the dwarf palm tree family, the Serenoa repens species specifically. It's found growing in various areas of the United States, as well as other countries. Extracts of SP contain standardized levels of active compounds, which are fatty acids and sterols which are believed to have the desired effects.

What is it supposed to do?

SP has been used for centuries to improve sperm production, increase breast size, improve sexual vigor, as well as to improve the symptoms of benign prostatic hyperplasia (BPH). Saw Palmetto extract is often recommended as a cure all for everything from hair loss (MPB) to benign prostate enlargement (BPH) to gynecomastia. Saw Palmetto is commonly added to various supplement formulas or sold alone. It's particularly popular with companies selling "andro" products who claim the added Saw Palmetto (SP) will block any possible negative effects the androstenedione, androstenediol, etc., might cause. As andro supplements are now banned, at least in the US, it's a moot point these days.

For non-athletes, Saw Palmetto, often combined with other herbs, has been a standard alternative treatment for BPH, an affliction that many men suffer from as they age. Some people are also under the impression that Saw Palmetto works as an anti estrogen and will block the conversion of testosterone into estrogen avoiding gynecomastia, also known fondly in bodybuilding circles as "bitch tits."

What does the research say for athletic performance?

Perhaps Saw Palmetto's best known sales pitch to bodybuilders and other athletes is its supposed ability to prevent the conversion of testosterone to dihydrotestosterone (DHT). The story goes like this:

The "male hormone" testosterone converts to the more powerful androgen (DHT) via the enzyme 5–alpha–reductase (5ar). DHT is known to be an important factor in the development of several problems many men face such as the aforementioned male pattern baldness and BPH. So, finding something that blocks the 5ar enzyme should reduce the amount of DHT and said male problems should be improved or avoided (FYI, this is also how the drug Finasteride, name brand Proscar, works.). Of course it's a lot more complicated than that but (a) it's beyond the scope of this section, and (b) only science geeks like me need to know the information in the real world.

Anyway, Saw Palmetto has often been cited as an herb able to block the 5ar enzyme and is recommended to people losing their hair or suffering from BPH and/or is added to "andro" products to theoretically block any negative effects of such products. Sounds great, but is it true? A handful of in vitro (test tube) studies have suggested that in certain cells, Saw Palmetto inhibits both types of the 5ar enzyme. This effect was noncompetitive and uncompetitive vs. Finasteride which works as a competitive inhibitor on the 5ar enzyme. However, in vivo studies (i.e., studies using either animals or people actually ingesting SP) have generally failed to show Saw Palmetto reduced DHT system-wide as its major effect.

Recent studies did not find SP altered testosterone either. It appears SP must be working by a different mechanism then as a simple 5ar inhibitor. One of the best known effects of SP not related to blocking 5ar, was a study that showed SP actually blocked the uptake of both testosterone and DHT by approximately 40% in eleven different tissues that were tested. This information scared off a lot of people from using SP as the thought of having their testosterone blocked at the cell surface along with DHT did not seem like a good idea to most bodybuilders. The study did lead one to believe that part of the effect of SP is as an androgen receptor antagonist (i.e. it blocks the receptor that testosterone binds to at the surface of the cell) and this would not be what an athlete wants trying to gain muscle. Several studies appear to show SP acts at the level of the androgen receptor. So in theory, SP could actually hinder your hard work in the gym, but it's really theoretical at this time.

It's also possible that some of the effects of SP are unrelated to its effects on androgens (via blocking testosterone –> DHT and/or blocking androgen receptors). For example, research finds SP potentially blocks the inflammation. SP was found to block several key enzymes involved in the production of inflammatory promoters/regulators such as leukotriene (LT) B4 as well as others produced from arachidonic acid via these enzymes.

What this tells us is that SP may act as a potent anti-inflammatory rather than as a blocker of testosterone to DHT. Interestingly enough, It's been shown that infiltration of the prostate by inflammatory cells is a key etiologic factor involved in the development of BPH. Translated, the immune system is involved in benign prostate enlargement.

Actually the immune system also appears to be involved in MPB and that's an interesting angle being pursued by researchers in the field.

Finally, we come to the reputation of SP as some kind of anti-estrogen. This is perhaps the most interesting, yet potentially confusing, effect of SP. Several studies have suggested SP may exert some type of anti-estrogenic effect on prostate tissues. However, and this is a huge however, it does not tell the entire story.

Why? I'll get to it, but first we have to do a little side track. If you recall from the chapter on **Anti-estrogens**, I wrote that there are two ways to effect estrogen. You can a) block the receptor site; or b) you can inhibit the enzyme (known as an aromatase) that converts testosterone, androstenedione, etc., into estrogens. To recap: when a molecule fits into the receptor but does not send an estrogenic signal it is called an "antagonist" meaning it prevents or "blocks" estrogen from getting to the receptor but does not in itself act as an estrogen. Hence the term "estrogen blocker." When something can lock into the receptor and does act as an estrogen, that is activates the receptor to one degree or another, it's called an "agonist."

So far so good right? What most people do not realize is that many things will have what is known as "mixed" antagonist and agonist properties. Before you slap your head in confusion, let me explain. Just because something has anti-estrogenic effects on one tissue does not mean it will have that effect on all tissues. In fact, and quite common, a compound can actually be an anti-estrogen in one tissue while actually acting as an estrogen (i.e., increasing estrogenic effects) in others! Many things are known to have mixed antagonist and agonist properties.

Remember when I said Tamoxifen was an estrogen receptor antagonist? Tamoxifen is a drug shown to have just such "mixed" properties, that is it has agonist or antagonist effects depending on the tissue in question. In women, Tamoxifen has been shown to act as an estrogen antagonist (i.e. blocks the estrogen receptor) in breast tissue but actually acts as an estrogen agonist in uterine tissues which is why it's used to treat breast cancer but may increase rates of uterine cancer. You all starting to catch my drift here?

" So where the hell is Brink going with this and what on God's earth does it mean to the hard training bodybuilder?!" you ask. Here is the rub: Just because SP might have some anti-estrogenic effects on the prostate does not mean it will prevent gyno, body fat increases, etc., known to occur from increased levels of estrogen (whether from andro products, steroid use, age, etc.) in all tissues. Companies or people that say otherwise are misleading you. There is no research to date that shows SP can prevent gyno or any other estrogen related problems bodybuilders are concerned about except possibly in prostate tissue. I realize it took me a while to get to that point but the reader can appreciate the fact that without the proper background you would be forced to just take my word for it. Now you know better.

You might recall that I mentioned another way of reducing estrogen, and that is by inhibiting the aromatase enzyme that converts testosterone into estrogens. A compound that can have that effect is an "anti-aromatase." Many people make the mistake of thinking Tamoxifen is an anti-aromatase when it is not. A true anti-aromatase is the drug Arimidex (anastrozole). There are also several plant isoflavones that appear to have anti-aromatase activity in vitro (test tube) research but have yet to show this effect in animals or people, especially in the doses most people take them. All the research I have seen to date points to SP as working at the level of the receptor rather than inhibiting the aromatase enzyme, which is why I focused mostly on explaining the concept of receptor agonists, antagonists, and compounds with "mixed" effects. Capiche?

Finally, the research on SP's effects on BPH are much more convincing with several large recent trials finding it was equally effective as drugs prescribed for the same use. The vast majority of people reading this are interested in SP's claims of acting as an anti-estrogen or blocker of DHT production, vs. as a treatment for BPH, and that's why I focused on those effects over BPH. It should be noted however that the studies supporting the use of SP for BPH is much more compelling.

Whether Saw Palmetto inhibits 5ar, blocks the uptake of testosterone and DHT into the prostate, blocks estrogen at the receptor, or actually inhibits certain pro-inflammatory enzymes responsible for the etiology and formation of BPH, is not certain at this time. Perhaps it works by all those mechanisms.

What about real world athletic performance?

Since SP has been around a long time, I have gotten a great deal of feedback from users. To date, no one has grown new hair, or prevented gyno, or anything else from the use of SP. Some have claimed it made their gyno worse. The only positive feedback I have gotten was from men who used it for BPH.

Will Brink's Recommendation

There is no research that directly looked at SP for hair loss in men (i.e. MPB), nor is there any research that has directly shown Saw Palmetto can reduce the potential side effects of any of the andro products or steroids. So, companies selling SP and claiming it can cure any of these issues are working with more hype then reality. I have yet to meet one single person who has grown one single hair from using SP. Prevent gyno? Ditto for the gyno as far as real world feedback is concerned.

As mentioned above, where Saw Palmetto looks far more promising is in its effects on BPH. Studies using Saw Palmetto extract have shown positive effects on BPH symptoms. Though it is unclear exactly how Saw Palmetto improves the symptoms of BPH, there appears to be enough data and clinical evidence in favor of Saw Palmetto as a treatment for men who suffer from an enlargement of the prostate that is not cancerous. So, if you have BPH, SP does in fact look like worthwhile treatment and that has been confirmed by real world observations. So, as a bodybuilding supplement in general, SP gets a thumbs down. As a possible treatment for BPH, it gets a "might be worth a try" rating. Men with BPH who wish to try SP, the standard dose is to use a standardized extract; two capsules daily of 160 mg (or one capsule of 320 mg) containing 85-95% sterols and lipids.

References

Breu W, Hagenlocher M, Redl K, et al. Anti-inflammatory activity of sabal fruit extracts prepared with supercritical carbon dioxide. In vitro antagonists of cyclooxygenase and 5–lipoxygenase metabolism. Arzneimittelforschung. 1992 Apr;42(4):547-51.

Casarosa C, Cosci di Coscio M, Fratta M. Lack of effects of a lyposterolic extract of Serenoa repens on plasma levels of testosterone, follicle–stimulating hormone, and luteinizing hormone. Clin Ther. 1988;10(5):585-8.

Delos S, Carsol JL, Ghazarossian E, et al. Testosterone metabolism in primary cultures of human prostate epithelial cells and fibroblasts. J Steroid Biochem Mol Biol. 1995 Dec;55(3-4):375-83.

Delos S, Iehle C, Martin PM, Raynaud JP. Inhibition of the activity of 'basic' 5 alpha–reductase (type 1) detected in DU 145 cells and expressed in insect cells. J Steroid Biochem Mol Biol. 1994 Mar;48(4):347-52.

Di Silverio F, Flammia GP, Sciarra A, et al. Plant extracts in BPH. Minerva Urol Nefrol. 1993 Dec;45(4):143-9.

Di Silverio F, D'Eramo G, Lubrano C, et al. Evidence that Serenoa repens extract displays an antiestrogenic activity in prostatic tissue of benign prostatic hypertrophy patients. Eur Urol. 1992;21(4):309-14.

el–Sheikh MM, Dakkak MR, Saddique A. The effect of Permixon on androgen receptors. Acta Obstet Gynecol Scand. 1988;67(5):397-9.

Iehle C, Delos S, Guirou O, Tate R, Raynaud JP, Martin PM. Human prostatic steroid 5 alpha–reductase isoforms—a comparative study of selective inhibitors. J Steroid Biochem Mol Biol. 1995 Sep;54(5-6):273-9.

Palin MF, Faguy M, LeHoux JG, Pelletier G. Inhibitory effects of Serenoa repens on the kinetic of pig prostatic microsomal 5alpha–reductase activity. Endocrine. 1998 Aug;9(1):65-9.

Paubert–Braquet M, Richardson FO, Servent–Saez N, et al. Effect of Serenoa repens extract (Permixon) on estradiol/testosterone–induced experimental prostate enlargement in the rat. Pharmacol Res. 1996 Sep–Oct;34(3-4-):171-9.

Paubert–Braquet M, Mencia Huerta JM, Cousse H, Braquet P. Effect of the lipidic lipidosterolic extract of Serenoa repens (Permixon) on the ionophore A23187–stimulated production of leukotriene B4 (LTB4) from human polymorphonuclear neutrophils. Prostaglandins Leukot Essent Fatty Acids. 1997 Sep;57(3):299-304.

Pytel YA, Vinarov A, Lopatkin N, et al. Long–term clinical and biologic effects of the lipidosterolic extract of Serenoa repens in patients with symptomatic benign prostatic hyperplasia. Adv Ther. 2002 Nov–Dec;19(6):297-306.

Strauch G, Perles P, Vergult G, et al. Comparison of finasteride (Proscar) and Serenoa repens (Permixon) in the inhibition of 5–alpha reductase in healthy male volunteers. Eur Urol. 1994;26(3):247-52.

Sultan C, Terraza A, Devillier C, et al. Inhibition of androgen metabolism and binding by a liposterolic extract of "Serenoa repens B" in human foreskin fibroblasts. J Steroid Biochem. 1984 Jan;20(1):515-9.

Wilt TJ, Ishani A, Stark G, et al. Saw palmetto extracts for treatment of benign prostatic hyperplasia: a systematic review. JAMA. 1998 Nov 11;280(18): 1604-9.

☥

Chapter

10

PROHORMONES
&
DESIGNER STEROIDS

The reader will note one section is lacking in this book, which is a the coverage of either prohormones or the more recent—and both now illegal for sale in the U.S,—"designer supplements." Prohormones such as M1T. 1–Test, 1–AD, etc. are a moot issue at this point due to the fact these products are basically unavailable and illegal.

Thus, there is no reason to cover the prohormones or "designer steroids" that followed.

After the banning of prohormones, it created a market for other products some call "designer supplements" which should really be called "designer steroids." I am of course talking about products such as Halodrol, Methyl–1–P, Methyl Masteron, PheraPlex, Trenadrol, and Superdrol, which were probably the most popular of the group prior to being banned for legal sale. Superdrol and the ilk have taken up where prohormones left off, bringing with them a new set of problems.

What are they you ask? Designer steroids (DS) existed in a very "gray area" of the law for a time . The most effective ones, such as

Superdrol, were simply true anabolic/androgenic steroids (AAS) that have been modified to be orally bioavailable.

Superdrol, for example was allegedly Masteron, with a methyl group attached to the C–17 (alpha) position (this "17–alpha–alkyl" modification is common to oral AAS, and is toxic to the liver, which is why supps like milk thistle, etc. were often a part of the cycles for orals modified in this fashion). Other DS based on well-known AAS:

– Trenadol, is—as you might have guessed—allegedly based on trenbolone.
– Halodrol—which has been withdrawn from the market—was based on Turinabol.

Other examples exist, but the above gives a sample of this group of products that existed after prohormones were banned. The reader will note I don't refer to them as "supplements" as they are nowhere near the definition of a supplement.

I know what you're thinking, "but Will, anabolic steroids are illegal, so how did they sell these products as supplements?" As I mentioned earlier, they fell into a grey area of the law. Relating to the legal aspect, I spoke to Rick Collins (www.steroidlaw.com) who is probably the foremost legal expert on steroids and the law. He told me:

" ...loopholes and poor language in the current Anabolic Steroid Control Act may not allow the government to treat and prosecute these products as anabolic steroids (although they may violate other laws). As expected, banning the true prohormones marketed until January only led to more aggressive and potentially more dangerous gray market "supplements"

The bottom line here, is that I did not recommend the use of these "supplements" when they were legal, and I don't now. They are modified versions of existing compounds/hormonal analogs, and we don't know their pharmacology in terms of efficacy, side effects, etc. A certain amount can be figured out from the chemistry (e.g., it's potential to convert to estradiol, the steroid it's derived from etc.) but make no mistake, small changes in hormones and hormone analogs can have profound changes on their pharmacology that are not discovered from a simple look at their molecular structure.

Make no doubt about this, the "designer supplements" were NOT prohormones but true designer steroids of unknown pharmacology. For that reason alone, I recommended people avoid them. Now that they are no longer legal OTC, even more so! If you happen to find some being sold on the 'net by some company attempting to fly under the radar, or perhaps in another country, etc. avoid! You are not using any sort of normal prohormone, but a true designer steroid with all the known—and more important—unknown effects good and bad. When they were legal, side effects typical of some AAS have been reported, such as elevated liver enzymes, hair loss, and increases in blood pressure. Some seem to be more effective then others as far as AAS like effects in terms of increased strength and muscle mass.

I was never a big fan of the prohormones when they were legal either, not because I thought they were particularly dangerous per se, but just not particularly effective for their intended use, and lacked any solid data in terms of both efficacy and safety.

This not being a steroid book, I will end the discussion there.

So what can be concluded from all this?

Although interest has died down substantially (since they're no longer being openly advertised and promoted), some are still buying and using DS from some black market sources usually via the 'net.

Legit supplement companies wisely have withdrawn such products from their line up since the ban, which is a good thing in my view.

I apologize to the reader for the ambiguous coverage of pro-hormones and DS's, but I have only added this section for those curious about them vs. any "how to" guide. They were not recommended for use when they were legal, much less now!

Ⴔ

Chapter

11

MAKING SENSE OF SUPPLEMENTS

T his chapter will attempt to help the reader categorize supplements in a way that helps them to prioritize what's clearly worth using, what "may be worth a try" and what's clearly not worth using, at least if adding strength, muscle mass, or improved performance is the goal. **The Supplement Scorecard** in the next chapter summarizes which supplements might be worth taking, and how much to take.

GAIN TWENTY POUNDS OF MUSCLE
LOSE FIFTY POUNDS OF FAT!

"Gain twenty pounds of muscle," "lose fifty pounds of fat," and "increase strength by a million percent" are the exaggerated headlines of the ads you find in most magazines and even some websites.

Certain supplements will help you gain muscle, lose fat, and increase strength, but as some people have found out the hard way, there are many supplements will do none of the above.

When it comes to training and diet, the average athlete has something of a semi-blueprint or plan as to how he or she will workout and eat. When it comes to supplements however, there is more of a hit-or-miss mentality with unrelated products being mixed together in the hope that something – *anything* – will happen to improve one's lean mass, body fat levels or health.

This can be a rather expensive and confusing process which can leave the person frustrated, poor, and just plain sour on the prospect of trying anything new for supplements. For example, you have Bob who is taking ribose, vitamin E, and L–carnitine. Then there is his training partner Joe who is taking L–arginine, CEE, and MCT oil. Bob's girlfriend uses soy protein, HMB, and chromium picolinate. Lets not forget Joe's girlfriend's friend Lisa who takes ginseng, CLA, and wild yam extract! Does this scenario seem oddly familiar to you?

The bottom line is that there are few black and white areas in the field nutrient supplementation, but also there is a whole lot of gray!

THE SUPPLEMENT PYRAMID

I tend to see supplements as a pyramid, and without a good foundation, you stand little chance of going to the next tier of your training goals.

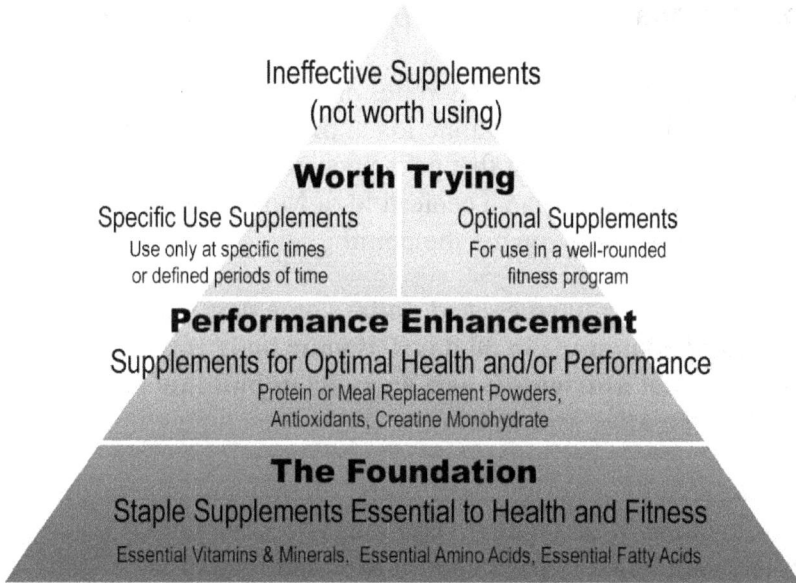

Ineffective Supplements
(not worth using)

Worth Trying

Specific Use Supplements
Use only at specific times
or defined periods of time

Optional Supplements
For use in a well-rounded
fitness program

Performance Enhancement

Supplements for Optimal Health and/or Performance
Protein or Meal Replacement Powders,
Antioxidants, Creatine Monohydrate

The Foundation

Staple Supplements Essential to Health and Fitness
Essential Vitamins & Minerals, Essential Amino Acids, Essential Fatty Acids

THE SUPPLEMENT PYRAMID

In my opinion, there are the supplements you should take all the time which are a staple part of the diet (the bottom of the pyramid).

Next, there are the supplements you can take regularly to improve performance, health, and/or convenience (the middle of the pyramid) but you can cycle these products or change them. Even though they are not necessarily essential to your health, they are clearly worth using on a regular basis.

Then there two more categories that have to be added; supplements that are useful only at specific times or for defined periods of time, and supplements that could be considered strictly optional, but have some use in a well rounded program. Within this group, there are also the supplements you can give an honest try and see if they work for you, but should not be relied on as foundation type supplements, and of these would form a sub category within the pyramid you see above.

Finally, there is the huge category of crap supplements not ever worth bothering with regardless of the application.

Foundational Supplements (the bottom of the pyramid)

Every single cell in your body relies on some vitamin, mineral, or other essential molecule to function at peak levels. A deficiency in a single essential nutrient that goes uncorrected will shut down the anabolic drive faster than a centerfold of Monica Brant gives the average guy a...well you get the point!

Why spend your hard earned dollars on a new supplement that promises "30 pounds in 30 days" if your body is shunting what little essential nutrients it gets away from building muscle to keeping you alive and well?

Obviously, a full description of every vitamin and mineral and all their functions would take several long and monotonous books to explain, so I won't even attempt it here, but I will give you an overview of how they're defined;

A foundational supplement is something you take year round and is usually an essential nutrient, such as a vitamin, mineral or fatty acid. Essential nutrients are just that—essential to life itself.

An essential nutrient is anything the body cannot manufacture itself and must be obtained from the diet or the person will get sick and/or perish if the nutritional deficiency is not corrected.

There are approximately 8 amino acids, 2 essential fatty acids, 13 vitamins, and 16 minerals that must be obtained from our diet on a regular basis and in adequate amounts or the human body will not function at its optimal capacity.

When I'm asked by an athlete what my opinion is of some new supplement, the conversation usually goes something like this: "Will, what do you think of this new product called Bull Gonad-Testomaxi-Bulk Up. Should I take it?" My answer is always something like "is your nutrition solid?" or "do you take a good multivitamin and multimineral? Are you taking fish oil and or flax oil or other oil blends (e.g., Udo's Choice™) and a good protein powder? Do you have the basics down?"

They give me a look of confusion and say "well no I'm not, but what does that have to do with the product I asked you about?" This is the equivalent of asking me if I like leg extensions out of the blue. I would ask "do you squat?" The point being, what reason is there to do leg extensions if a person does not do a foundational exercise such as the squat? There is no reason, unless your goal is legs of string!

Are you starting to see what I am getting at here? **What reason is there to even bother with a fancy new supplement if your essential nutrient needs are not being met?**

Another product that should be considered as a foundational, year round nutrient is a source of unprocessed and unaltered essential fatty acids. As with most vitamins and minerals, it is virtually impossible to get optimal amounts of unprocessed essential fatty acids (especially the omega–3 fatty acids) from our heavily processed food supply. The two essential fatty acids we need are Linoleic acid (LA) which is an omega–6 fatty acid, and Alpha–Linolenic acid (ALA) which is an omega–3 fatty acid. Unless you have been living in a cave for the past few years, you know the nutritional authorities "in the know" have been singing the praises of these amazing fatty acids for some time now.

This is the point where we could (and maybe should?) get into that ongoing argument by mainstream nutritionists and doctors who say "you get all the vitamins you need from your food" or "supplements just give you expensive urine."

It depends on the nutrient in question, but bottom line is this; the chances of a strength training athlete getting optimal (as opposed to adequate) amounts of vitamins, minerals, and essential fatty acids from our nutrient deficient processed food supply is zero, zip, nada - ain't gonna happen!

I realize it has taken an amazingly long time to just get to the point of this section, which is that you should always be taking a good multivitamin everyday of your life. Although this seems like common sense, you would be amazed at how many athletes don't take them, assuming they get all they need from those nine chicken breasts and three boxes of white rice they eat every day...

And the last time I checked, chemotherapy, cholesterol medications, heart bypass operations, and countless other avoidable medical treatments are considerably more expensive than the average multivitamin and mineral supplement.

Performance Enhancement Supplements (2nd row of the pyramid)

WHEY PROTEIN: Unlike vitamins, minerals, and essential fatty acids, adequate amounts of essential and non-essential amino acids can be gotten from our food. However, getting all the amino acids we need from our food is not always convenient and it is arguable whether or not we can get optimal amounts for muscle growth from our foods; as opposed to adequate amounts.

Also, several protein foods have specific amino acids or properties that we want as athletes. For example, whey protein has the highest biological value (BV), is almost 50% essential amino acids, and is moderately high in glutamine (though some companies add more glutamine).

Besides being a great protein period, whey protein improves immunity and raises glutathione, to mention only a few potential health benefits. Thus, a good protein supplement or high quality meal replacement product is an important part of any well planned supplement program, although you don't need it per se and could live without such products if you had to.

ANTIOXIDANTS: Without going into a long and mega boring biochemical explanation, antioxidants are a special class of vitamins and other non vitamin compounds that neutralize free radicals. Free radical pathology has been implicated in a broad range of diseases such as cancer, atherosclerosis, immune deficiency, and diabetes, to name only a few afflictions we would all like to avoid. More important to athletes, free radicals cause inflammation, damage to muscle fibers, fatigue, and possibly immune suppression.

Intense exercise causes a dramatic rise in free radicals with a simultaneous reduction in antioxidant systems within the body to fight them. If left unchecked, free radicals will lead to the breakdown of muscle tissue and various other problems, and we sure as hell don't want that! Antioxidants are just not all that sexy and at times don't get as much attention as they should, but I can assure you they are very important nutrients for long term health and continued progress in making gains in muscle. While no one ever exploded with new muscle from the simple addition of antioxidants to their diet, they may help build muscle in the long run as well as improve immunity to a variety of challenges. Remember, you can't train if you're sick in bed!

Antioxidants have also been found to be somewhat liver protective from the use of oral steroids. Antioxidants such as vitamin E and C, and many others can be found in a good antioxidant formula and should be used year round by all hard training athletes of both the natural and non–natural variety.

CREATINE MONOHYDRATE: Though it may be the best thing since the discovery of sliced bread, creatine is not an essential nutrient. Certain foods (i.e., red meat) are moderately high in creatine and the body can synthesis creatine from the amino acids arginine, glycine, and methionine. Regardless of this fact, the intake of creatine in far higher amounts than could ever be found in food or synthesized in the body has been verified by the research and proven in the real world to put muscle on people and increase strength. It's cheap, it works, and it's safe, so this is definitely a year round performance supplement.

Creatine has also been found to have an amazing array of potential health benefits and may help with a vast number of diseases. For more information on that, download my recent report on the topic from www.creatine-report.com.

Optional but useful supplements that are worth trying (3rd row of the Pyramid)

These supplements are not as important as the ones in the previous two categories, but are nice additions to round out your supplement program.

OPTIONAL USE SUPPLEMENTS: This category comes under those supplements that "might be worth a try" and: (a) have some research behind them but more needs to be done, (b) seem to work for some people but not for others ,(c) are expensive, (d) the "experts" can't seem to agree on it, that is, some experts like the product(s) and some don't, or; (e) all of the above!

Many of these are all listed in **The Supplement Scorecard** in the next chapter. Clearly, I have my own feelings on which one of them are good or bad which you can see by how they were reviewed, but they all have at least some research behind them, appear to work for some people, and there are plenty of "experts" who would not agree with me if I were to tell you what I think of all of them.

The main point of this section is this; Although they might be worth a try, I would never recommend giving up or stopping the use of any of the supplements in the first two levels of the pyramid to use them. For example, you would never stop taking antioxidants to start taking glutamine or phosphatidylserine, or stop taking whey protein to start taking ZMA.

SPECIFIC USE SUPPLEMENTS: The supplements in this category cannot be classified as either good or bad, but they are useful at specific times and for specific purposes. Ephedrine comes to mind as the perfect example of a product in this category. Ephedrine is not something that should be taken year round in my view. Taken occasionally before a workout to give a person a boost, and the stuff works great for that reason. If taken for a defined period of time for a specific purpose, combined with caffeine, it is a fantastic and relatively safe way to reduce body fat.

Say you want to get lean for the summer. You clean up your diet a little, add in some extra aerobics and take an ephedrine/caffeine mixture for ten to twelve weeks. Voila! You're ripped and ready for summer. However, taking ephedrine year round is hard on the system, can have potential side effects, and will ultimately be counterproductive to adding muscle in the long run if not cycled on and off or used occasionally as energy booster for tough workouts. The problem is, I see people popping handfuls of the stuff every time they train all year round. That's a mistake.

Ineffective Supplements (4th row of the pyramid)

From bug molting hormones (beta–ecdysterone) to bee spit (bee pollen/royal jelly), this is a long, long, long (did I mention long?), list! Hmm, where do we start? Vanadyl sulfate? Plant sterols? Myostatin inhibitors? What can I say, there are a lot of worthless supplements out there in the world. See The Supplement Scorecard for a partial list.

THE SUPPLEMENT SCORECARD

This chapter is a summarization of the supplement recommendations in the reviews, and how they rank according to the framework in the Making Sense of Supplements chapter. This scorecard will help you choose the types and doses of supplements that will work best for you and help you make the best use of the money in your supplement budget.

FOUNDATIONAL SUPPLEMENTS

These are the elements that are part of the backbone of any solid supplementation program. If these bases aren't covered, additional supplements are likely to be a waste of time and money.

Multivitamin/Mineral Complex

Recommended Dose: At a minimum, a multivitamin should supply 100% of the RDA/DRI of the 13 major vitamins. A decent multi will also typically contain useful doses (25%-100%) of the major and trace minerals.

Essential Fatty Acids

Recommended Dose:

Flax Oil: 1 tablespoon per 75 lb body weight – or -
Udo's Choice™: 1 tablespoon per 50 lb body weight
Fish Oil: the equivalent amount needed for 2g EPA + DHA

φ

PERFORMANCE ENHANCEMENT SUPPLEMENTS

Supplements under this umbrella are some basic supplements that
will give you the most value for your money, and help enhance the
results of your workout/nutrition programs. Some of these
supplements are also used as a means of convenience, as in the case
of protein powders and creatine.

Whey Protein

Recommended Dose: 0.5 g/kg for pre9/post-workout; also as
needed to increase protein intake

Antioxidants

Recommended Dose: Vitamin C: 200-500 mg/day; Vitamin E: 400
IU/day

Creatine Monohydrate

Recommended Dose: Loading (if desired but not required): 5 g x 4 times per day for 5 days; otherwise, 3-5 g/day for 1 month, followed by 2-3 g/day for maintenance.

Note: Creatine monohydrate should be properly dissolved before consuming; using a warm liquid is recommended.

☧

SUPPLEMENTS THAT ARE OPTIONAL, BUT CAN BE USEFUL FOR A MUSCLE BUILDING PROGRAM

These supplements are not essentials, but can provide some additional benefits.

Beta–Alanine

Recommended Dose: 3-6 g/day in divided doses

Glutamine

Recommended Dose: 5-20 g, usually taken post-workout

Taurine

Recommended Dose: Therapeutic doses range from ~1.5 g-6 g/day

Tyrosine

Recommended Dose: 0.5-2 g, taken on an empty stomach

Phosphatidylserine

Recommended Dose: 400-800 mg/day

Casein

Recommended Dose: Use as needed/desired for additional protein (not recommended for pre-/post-workout)

☧

OTHER PROTEINS

Note: for most people, some supplemental whey and casein should be sufficient. However, you may want to use other sources in the event of allergy and/or intolerance, or simply for the sake of variety.

Egg White Protein

Recommended Dose: Use as needed/desired for additional protein (not recommended for pre-/post-workout)

Serum Protein Isolate

Recommended Dose: Use as needed/desired for additional protein (not recommended for pre-/post-workout)

Vegetarian Proteins (Soy, Hemp, Rice)

Recommended Dose: Use as needed/desired for additional protein (not recommended for pre-/post-workout)

ϕ

SUPPLEMENTS TO EXPERIMENT WITH OR MIGHT BE WORTH A TRY

The evidence for these supplements is mixed and inconclusive, but some people have found them useful

Citrulline

Recommended Dose: A minimum of 6 g/day-can be in divided doses (i.e., 3 g x 2x/day

Colostrum

Recommended Dose: 20 g/day

Bacopa Monnieri

Recommended Dose: 200-400 mg of an extract standardized to 20% bacosides

Ashwagandha

Recommended Dose: 3-6g/day of the dried root, or 300-500mg of a standardized extract

Cordyceps

Recommended Dose: 1-4 g/day of a preparation standardized to contain 5%-7% cordycepic acid

Ginseng

Recommended Dose: 50-100 mg per day of an extract containing at least 7%-10% ginsenosides, 2-3 times per day

Rhodiola Rosea

Recommended Dose: 100-200 mg of an extract standardized to 3% rosavins

ф

SUPPLEMENTS USEFUL FOR SPECIFIC APPLICATIONS

The supplements in this group are most useful for specific situations, such as cutting or pre-workout

BCAAs

Recommended Dose: 5-10 g/day in divided doses

Caffeine

Recommended Dose: 100-200 mg pre-workout (do not take within 4 hours of bedtime)

CLA

Recommended Dose: 3-6 g/day in divided doses

ɸ

SUPPLEMENTS THAT ARE UNPROVEN OR INEFFECTIVE

Although not useful for as a "sports supplement" (i.e., they don't appear to improve strength, LBM, or performance) that does not mean they don't have other potential benefits. Readers should consult the individual supplement reviews for further information on each in terms of potential benefits not directly related to sports applications.

Unproven or Ineffective Sports Supplements

* in addition to what is obtained through diet or general multivitamin/mineral supplement

7–Keto–DHEA	Glycerol
Agmatine	HMB/KIC
Arachidonic Acid	Horny Goat Weed
Arginine/AAKG	I3C/DIM
ATD	Maca
Avena Sativa	MCTs
Beta–Sitosterol	Methoxyisoflavone
Calcium*	Myostatin Inhibitors

Unproven or Ineffective Sports Supplements

* in addition to what is obtained through diet
or general multivitamin/mineral supplement

Carnitine	Ornithine/OKG
Chromium Picolinate*	Resveratrol
Cissus Quadrangularis	Ribose
Chrysin	Saw Palmetto
DHEA	Tongkat Ali
Ecdysterones	Tribulus Terrestris
Fenugreek (Testofen)	Urtica Dioica
GABA	Vanadyl Sulphate*
GH Supplements	ZMA

USING THE SUPPLEMENT SCORECARD

To illustrate how the Scorecard can be used to evaluate a supplement, we'll apply the information to a commercial product that I'll call "Mega-Test Xtreme" for the purposes of this discussion. Mega-Test Xtreme is based on an actual supplement.

Let's take a look at the ingredients and dosage instructions:

Serving Size: 2 Capsules
Servings Per Container: 30

Amount Per Serving:
Zinc (Chelate): 30 mg 200%
Vitamin B6: 5 mg 200%
Magnesium (Aspartate): 100 mg 20%
Tribulus Terrestris Extract: 40% 900 mg
Dehydroepiandrosterone (DHEA): 50 mg
Test Support Blend: 550 mg
    Avena sativa Extract
    Peruvian Maca Root
    Eurycoma longifolia Jack Extract
    Saw Palmetto Berry Extract
    Chrysin

The first 3 ingredients are: zinc, vitamin B6 and magnesium. Recognize it? It's the same combination of nutrients that you get in

ZMA, which is in the worth a try table. If you look a little closer though, you'll see that the amounts are different.

According to the table, a serving of ZMA provides: 30 mg zinc (as monomethionine/aspartate).

- This supplement provides the standard amount of zinc, although it doesn't specify what it's chelated to. Still, we can let that slide, since there's no real proof that the form used in ZMA is more bioavailable than other forms.

- 450 mg magnesium (as aspartate). There's a big difference here: Mega-Test Xtreme provides only 100 mg of magnesium (aspartate).

- 10.5 mg vitamin B6. Another difference—our example supplement contains 5 mg of vitamin B6 , which is less than half the amount in ZMA.

So these ingredients have the "feel" of ZMA, but don't quite match up to the real thing. Do the differences matter? It's hard to say, but since magnesium is something that athletes are short on, and I'd want to make sure I was getting an adequate amount in my diet, I would be concerned about this.

The next ingredient is **Tribulus Terrestris Extract: 40%**. Presumably, this means that the extract has been standardized to 40% of a particular compound, but what it might be isn't stated. This isn't likely to matter though, since there's no evidence that Tribulus even works—which is why it's on the **Ineffective** list.

Then there's **Dehydroepiandrosterone (DHEA): 50 mg**. While DHEA is ineffective in terms of sports applications, if you're middle aged or older, there's a good chance that your DHEA levels might be low, which means it may indeed have health benefits to you. So DHEA is a supplement that might be worthwhile to take, and something that you should put in the optional list, albeit for other reasons than adding mass/strength.

Finally, we have a proprietary blend that contains several different herbal extracts:

- Avena sativa: this is on the **Ineffective** list, and for good reason. There is exactly zero good evidence that it has any effects at all on testosterone.

- Peruvian Maca root: this is also on the **Ineffective** list. The one small positive study discussed in the review noted that 1.5-3.0 grams were used. There are only 550 mg in this entire herbal blend. So even if maca were effective, the dose here is too small.

- Eurycoma longifolia Jack Extract: also **Ineffective** for raising testosterone and/or enhancing lean mass/strength.

- Saw Palmetto berry extract: SP has some use for BPH, but in larger doses than this 550 mg blend could possibly provide. It's also on the **Ineffective** list.

- Chrysin: also **Ineffective** since it's not well absorbed.

Mega-Test Xtreme provides a few compounds that might be useful for health reasons, but most of the ingredients will do nothing to boost testosterone, or increase muscle mass.

Verdict? Save your money!

Other supplements can be a bit tougher to evaluate. Take a rival product, "Ultra T-Boost," for example:

Serving Size: 1 Tablet
Servings Per Container: 30

Amount Per Serving:
Niacin 30 mg 150%
Zinc (as zinc oxide) 30 mg 200%
Copper (as copper oxide) 4mg 200%
Premium Blend: 541 mg
 Korean Ginseng root 10:1 extract
 Ginkgo Biloba leaf standardized extract
 Tribulus Terrestris extract (45% saponins)(aerial)
 L–Arginine HCl
 Avena Sativa extract (aerial parts)
 Horny Goat Weed standardized extract (whole plant)
 Maca Root
 Muira Puama extract (aerial part)
 Octacosanol
 Saw Palmetto berry
 Swedish Flower Pollen extract

Once again, there are ingredients that are on the **Ineffective and Unproven List**: Tribulus terrestris, Avena sativa, arginine, horny goat weed, maca, and saw palmetto.

Niacin, zinc, and copper are essential nutrients, but—as noted in the previous example—you should already have these covered. Ginseng is on the **Supplements to Experiment With** list. So far, so good.

But there are some other ingredients that aren't anywhere to be found in the Scorecard: Gingko biloba, Muira puama, octocosanol, and Swedish flower pollen extract. What to do?

First, a reality check; it would be virtually impossible for me to cover every single ingredient ever included in the thousands of supplements marketed to athletes. For one thing, many have nothing to do with adding muscle, but are fat burners, mood enhancers, etc. Others are not widely used. So it would be a waste of space to cover things like Urtica dioca, Saraparilla, Kudzu extract, Ajuga turkestanica, "moomiyo", etc.

This book attempts to cover the major, and minor supplements sold to athletes, but can't cover everything known to mankind!

See You In The Gym!

ȹ

For More Information

For more information, check out the companion web site to this book:

http://www.thesportssupplementbible.com

There you will find free reports, additional articles, videos, and other resources that will help you save money, and stop the wasted time on potentially worthless supplements!

Also see the other links below to get additional information.

INFORMATION ON SUPPLEMENTS

http://www.creatine-report.com

http://www.BrinkZone.com

STUDIES AND OTHER SCIENTIFIC DATA

http://www.ncbi.nlm.nih.gov/pubmed/

φ

INDEX

(-)

(–)–3,4–divanillyltetrahydrofuran, 225

1

1,2,3–propanetriol
glycerol, 286

1,3,7–trimethylxanthine
Caffeine, 261

3

3,5,4'–trihydroxystilbene
Resveratrol, 212

5

5,7–dihydroxyflavone
Chrysin, 181

5–methyl–7–methoxy–isoflavone
methoxy, 235

6

6–OXO, 176, 177, 179, 188, 189, 190

7

7–Keto DHEA
DHEA, 76, 77, 78

A

acetyl–L–carnitine
Carnitine, 68, 69

Agmatine, 49, 51, 52, 53, 327

AIDS
HIV, 132, 294

alpha–ketoisocaproic acid, 85, 86, 87, 89

Alpha–lactalbumin, 125

alpha–linolenic acid
ALA, 121, 143, 145, 146, 157, 158

amino acids, 12, 13, 19, 24, 25, 26, 31, 36, 37, 40, 42, 59, 68, 85, 88, 102, 103, 113, 125, 126, 127, 133, 272, 280, 281, 282, 286, 314, 316, 317

androst–4–ene–3,6,17–trione
6–OXO, 188, 189, 191

antagonist, 175, 178, 179, 213, 261, 300, 301, 302

anti-cancer, 73, 129, 185, 229, 235, 253, 275

anti-estrogen, 175, 176, 177, 188, 301, 302, 303

antioxidant, 120, 123, 126, 127, 148, 163, 165, 166, 167, 169, 181, 194, 205, 208, 214, 235, 239, 242, 243, 245, 246, 248, 253, 257, 268, 275, 317

Arachidonic Acid, 54, 327

arginine–alpha–ketoglutarate
AAKG, 14

Ashwagandha, 239, 240, 241, 242, 243, 325

ATD
3,17–dioxo–etiochol–1,4,6–triene, 176, 177, 178, 179, 180, 327

Avena sativa, 194, 196, 331, 332

avenacosides, 194

avenanthramides, 194

Ayurvedic medicine, 239, 270

B

Bacopa extracts. See Bacopa monnieri

Bacopa monnieri
Brahmi, 243, 244, 245, 246

BCAAs, 24, 25, 85, 112, 326
See Branched Chain Amino Acids

Beta2–microglobulin, 125

Beta–Alanine, 19, 322

beta–glucan, 194, 196

beta–hydroxymethylbutyric acid.
See HMB

Beta–lactoglobulin, 125

beta–sitosterol, 228

biotin, 135

bitch tits. See gynecomastia

Bovine Serum Albumin, 125

Bovine Spongiform Encephalitis.
See Mad Cow Disease

Branched Chain Amino Acids
BCAAs, 24

C

caffeine, 36, 44, 45, 261, 262, 263, 264,
265, 266, 272, 273, 319

Calcium, 135, 137, 139, 327

cancer, 76, 125, 143, 168, 169, 175,
184, 185, 186, 187, 202, 212, 213,
214, 227, 228, 229, 230, 275, 278,
294, 302, 317

Cannabis, 121

cardiovascular disease, 17, 212, 269

cardiovascular health, 120, 274

Carnitine, 68, 69, 328

Casein, 101, 106, 323

catabolic, 24, 35, 54, 55, 85, 91, 101,
105, 106, 143, 144, 152, 172, 229,
238, 282, 291, 295

Chloride, 135

Chocamine
Cocoa Extract, 272, 273

cholesterol medications, 316

Chromium, 135, 140, 141, 142, 144,
153, 328

chrysin, 181, 182, 183, 235

cis–9, trans–11 isomer, 275

Cissus extract, 269

Cissus quadrangularis, 268, 269, 270,
271

Citrulline, 27, 28, 29, 30, 324

CLA
Conjugated Linoleic Acid, 275, 276,
277, 278, 312, 326

cobalamin
B12, 135

Cocoa, 272, 273, 274
See Chocamine

Colostrum, 108, 109, 111, 324

conalbumin, 112

Conjugated Linoleic Acid
CLA, 275, 279

copper, 272, 332

Copper, 135, 173

Cordyceps, 248, 249, 250, 251, 258,
325

creatine, 12, 14, 19, 20, 22, 23, 59, 60,
61, 62, 63, 64, 65, 66, 87, 96, 127,
132, 264, 265, 266, 267, 317, 318,
321, 334

Creatine Monohydrate, 59, 317, 322
See creatine

Cystoseira canariensis, 296, 297

D

designer steroids, 307, 309

DHEA, 72, 73, 74, 75, 76, 77, 78, 200, 201, 327, 328, 330

DHEA–S
DHEA–sulphate, 72, 74

DHT
dihydrotestosterone, 213, 225, 227, 228, 230, 299, 300, 301, 303

DIM
diindolylmethane, 184, 185, 186, 327

D–ribose. See Ribose

E

ecdysterone
beta–ecdysterone, 232, 233, 319

Egg White Protein, 112, 323

essential amino acids, 13, 316

essential fatty acids
EFA's, 58, 134, 143, 144, 145, 147, 148, 149, 291, 314, 315, 316

Essential fatty acids
EFA's, 136

estrogen, 76, 77, 174, 175, 176, 177, 178, 180, 181, 182, 184, 185, 186, 187, 188, 189, 190, 199, 212, 213, 229, 299, 301, 302, 303

estrogen antagonist, 175, 302

estrogen blocker, 175, 301

F

fatty acids, 54, 68, 90, 91, 143, 144, 145, 146, 152, 153, 157, 158, 279, 286, 290, 291, 299, 315

Fenugreek
Trigonella foenum–graecum, 198, 199, 200, 201, 328

Finasteride, 300

fish oil, 145, 146, 150, 152, 153, 154, 155, 156, 158, 315

Fish Oil. See EFA's, See EFA's

flax oil, 143, 145, 146, 147, 148, 149, 150, 152, 292, 315
See EFA's

Fluoride, 135

folic acid, 135

Foundational Supplements, 314, 320

Fructose, 94

G

GABA, 80, 81, 82, 83, 84, 328

gamma–aminobutyric acid, 83, 84
See GABA

GH
Growth Hormone, 15, 16, 32, 36, 37, 49, 51, 80, 81, 82, 84, 133, 280, 281, 282, 283, 284, 285, 328

ginseng, 209, 239, 252, 253, 254, 255, 312

globulins, 112

glucose intolerance, 239

glucose tolerance, 162, 199, 264

Glutamine, 31, 33, 322

glutathione
GSH, 126, 131, 133, 166, 240, 316

glycerol, 90, 286, 287, 288, 289

glycerol consumption, 287

glycerol monostearate, 288

glycine, 59, 70, 86, 126, 317

Glycomacropeptides, 125

green tea extract, 269

gynecomastia
bitch tits, 188, 299

H

Halodrol, 307, 308

Hemp, 121
  See Cannabis

hemp protein, 120, 121, 123

HGH
  Human Growth Hormone, 280

HIV, 60, 125, 133, 212, 294, 297

HMB, 85, 86, 87, 88, 89, 217, 312, 327

Horny Goat Weed
  licentious goat-fire, 204, 327

I

I3C, 184, 185, 186, 327
  Indole–3–carbinol, 184

IGF–1, 35, 40, 49, 73, 108, 109, 115,
  116, 170, 172, 280, 284

Immunoglobulins, 125

in vitro, 50, 52, 55, 77, 83, 145, 161,
  177, 181, 183, 184, 190, 194, 195,
  197, 204, 205, 220, 225, 243, 249,
  257, 268, 275, 294, 296, 300, 303

insulin sensitivity, 41, 42, 43, 75, 143,
  144, 152, 161, 198, 248, 250, 251,
  262, 263, 264, 265, 266, 275, 277

Iodine, 135

Iron, 135

isoflavones, 235, 236, 303

K

KIC, 85, 86, 87, 89, 327
  See alpha–ketoisocaproic acid

L

Lactoferrin, 125

Lactoperoxidase, 125

L–arginine
  Arginine, 14, 18, 53, 312

L–carnitine–L–tartrate
  Carnitine, 68, 69

L–cysteine, 126

LDL–cholesterol, 120

Lepidium meyenii
  Maca, 209, 211

Leucine.
  See L–leucine

L–glutamine, 31, 126

L–Glutamine
  Glutamine, 31

linoleic acid
  LA, 54, 56, 143, 208, 275, 278, 279

L–leucine, 24, 85, 86

long chain fatty acids, 290

Long Jack, 215
  See Tongkat Ali

L–serine, 90

L–Tyrosine
  Tyrosine, 44

lysozyme, 112, 128

Lysozyme, 125

M

Maca, 209, 210, 211, 327, 331

Mad Cow Disease, 91, 115

magnesium, 63, 64, 121, 170, 171, 272,
  329, 330

Magnesium, 135, 173

Manganese, 135

MCTs
  Medium Chain Triglycerides, 290,
  291, 292, 327

Medium Chain Triglycerides. See , See

Metabolic Syndrome, 263

metabolites, 12, 14, 27, 47, 53, 54, 55, 56, 78, 79, 85, 173, 184, 185, 187, 226, 278

methoxyisoflavone
5–methyl–7–methoxy–isoflavone, 235

Methyl Masteron, 307

Methyl–1–P, 307

Molybdenum, 135

multimineral, 315

multivitamin, 170, 171, 315, 316, 320, 327

muscular dystrophy, 60, 294

Myostatin
Myostatin Inhibitors, 294, 295, 297, 319, 327

myostatin inhibitors, 294

N

niacin/niacinamide
B3, 135

nitric oxide
NO, 14, 17, 18, 27, 36, 37, 38, 39, 49, 52, 53, 195, 196, 205, 207, 208

O

omega–3, 56, 57, 58, 121, 143, 144, 145, 146, 148, 149, 152, 153, 154, 155, 156, 315

Omega–3.
See EFAs

Omega–3 lipids, 144, 153, 156

omega–6, 54, 56, 57, 58, 121, 143, 144, 148, 149, 315

Ornithine, 35, 37, 38, 328

Ornithine alpha–ketoglutarate
OKG, 35, 37, 38

Ornithine Alpha–Ketoglutarate (OKG), 35

ovalbumin, 112, 251

ovomucin, 112

ovomucoid, 112

P

PDCAAS
Protein Digestibility Corrected Amino Acid Score, 120, 121, 122

Performance Enhancement Supplements, 316, 321

phenylethylamine, 272, 273

PheraPlex, 307

Phosphatidylserine, 90, 93, 323

Phosphorus, 135

phytoecdysteroids, 232

phytosterols, 228, 231

plant steroids, 232

polyphenols, 272, 273

Potassium, 135

prohormones, 180, 307, 308, 309

propionyl–L–carnitine
Carnitine, 68, 69

Protein powder, 99

R

resveratrol, 212, 213, 214

Rhodiola extract, 256

Rhodiola rosea, 250, 256, 257, 258

riboflavin
B2, 135

Ribose, 94, 96, 97, 328

rice protein, 120, 122, 123

rosavins, 256, 257, 325

S

Saw Palmetto, 178, 299, 300, 303, 304, 328, 331

Selenium, 135

Serum Protein Isolate, 115, 324

Sodium, 135

soy protein, 118, 120, 121, 122, 123, 312

soy protein isolates, 120

stinging nettle
Urtica dioica, 224, 225, 226

Sucrose, 94

sugar, 77, 94, 141, 159, 161, 198, 199, 253, 272

sulfated polysaccharides, 296

Sulfur, 135

Superdrol, 307, 308

Syndrome X, 144, 153, 263

T

Tamoxifen, 175, 178, 302, 303

Taurine, 40, 42, 43, 322

Testofen™, 198, 200, 201

testosterone, 5, 49, 55, 63, 73, 75, 76, 77, 170, 171, 172, 173, 174, 175, 176, 177, 178, 179, 180, 181, 182, 184, 185, 186, 188, 189, 190, 192, 194, 195, 198, 199, 200, 201, 204, 206, 208, 210, 211, 213, 214, 215, 217, 218, 220, 222, 224, 225, 227, 228, 229, 230, 232, 235, 283, 299, 300, 301, 303, 305, 331

testosterone booster, 215

The Supplement Scorecard, 10, 311, 318, 319, 320

theobromine, 272, 273

thiamin
B1, 134, 135

Tongkat Ali, 215, 218, 328

Trenadrol, 307

Tribulus terrestris, 200, 220, 222, 223, 332

Tribulus Terrestris Extract, 330

Trigonella foenum–graecum L Fenurgreek, 198

tyramine, 272, 273, 274

U

Urtica dioica, 224, *See* stinging nettle

V

Vanadium, 159

Vanadyl Sulfate, 136

vanadyl sulphate, 160

Vegetarian Proteins
Soy, Hemp, Rice, 120, 123, 324

vitamin A
retinol/retinal/retinoic acid, 135

vitamin B6, 40, 80, 170, 329, 330

vitamin C
ascorbic acid, 134, 135, 148, 163, 164, 165, 166, 196, 229, 268

Vitamin C, 163, 164, 321

vitamin D
calcitriol, 135

vitamin E
tocopherols/tocotrienols, 121, 135, 149, 166, 167, 168, 291, 312, 317

Vitamin E, 166, 167, 321

vitamin K
menaquinone, 135

W

weight loss, 3, 44, 45, 68, 70, 72, 76, 77, 78, 105, 140, 141, 145, 146, 149, 154, 269, 271, 291

Whey Protein, 125, 316, 321

Z

Zinc, 135, 170, 173

ZMA, 136, 170, 171, 172, 173, 318, 328, 330

www.ingramcontent.com/pod-product-compliance
Lightning Source LLC
Chambersburg PA
CBHW070552270326
41926CB00013B/2289